The Natural Medicine Guide to

SCHIZOPHRENIA

Also by Stephanie Marohn

Natural Medicine First Aid Remedies

Other Titles in the Healthy Mind Guide Series:

The Natural Medicine Guide to Autism

The Natural Medicine Guide to Depression

The Natural Medicine Guide to Bipolar Disorder

The Natural Medicine Guide to Anxiety

The Natural Medicine Guide to

SCHIZOPHRENIA

Stephanie Marohn

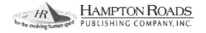

HAMPTON ROADS
PUBLISHING COMPANY, INC.

Cover design by Bookwrights Design
Cover art/photographic image © 2003 Loyd Chapplow
Interior illustrations Medi Clip Images © Williams
& Wilkins. All rights reserved.

Hampton Roads Publishing Company, Inc.
1125 Stoney Ridge Road
Charlottesville, VA 22902

434-296-2772
fax: 434-296-5096
e-mail: hrpc@hrpub.com
www.hrpub.com

If you are unable to order this book from your local
bookseller, you may order directly from the publisher.
Call 1-800-766-8009, toll-free.

Library of Congress Cataloging-in-Publication Data

Marohn, Stephanie.
 The natural medicine guide to schizophrenia / Stephanie Marohn.
   p. cm.
Includes bibliographical references and index.
  ISBN 1-57174-289-1
1. Schizophrenia--Alternative treatment. 2. Orthomolecular
therapy.
3. Naturopathy. I. Title.
  RC514.M358 2003
  616.89'806--dc21

                          2003014794

            ISBN 1-57174-289-1

          10 9 8 7 6 5 4 3 2 1

Printed on acid-free paper in Canada

THE HEALTHY 🌑 MIND GUIDES

THE HEALTHY MIND GUIDES are a series of books offering original research and treatment options for reversing or ameliorating several so-called mental disorders, written by noted health journalist and author Stephanie Marohn. The series' focus is the natural medicine approach, a refreshing and hopeful outlook based on treating individual needs rather than medical labels, and addressing the underlying imbalances—biological, psychological, emotional, and spiritual.

Each book in the series offers the very latest information about the possible causes of each disorder, and presents a wide range of effective, practical therapies drawn from extensive interviews with physicians and other practitioners who are innovators in their respective fields. Case studies throughout the books illustrate the applications of these therapies, and numerous resources are provided for readers who want to seek treatment.

The information in this book is not intended to replace medical care. The author and publisher disclaim responsibility for how you choose to employ the information in this book and the results or consequences of any of the treatments covered.

To Nijinsky, for all the dances that might have been

Acknowledgments

My deep gratitude to the doctors and other healing professionals who provided information on their work for the natural medicine treatment chapters in the book. I am very appreciative of all the time and energy you so generously gave. Specifically, my thanks to:

Johannes Beckmann, M.D.
Lina Garcia, D.D.S., D.M.D.
Abram Hoffer, M.D., Ph.D.
Dietrich Klinghardt, M.D., Ph.D.
Michael Lesser, M.D.
Judyth Reichenberg-Ullman, N.D., L.C.S.W.
Hugh D. Riordan, M.D.
Malidoma Patrice Somé, Ph.D.
William J. Walsh, Ph.D.

Appreciation to Sue Trowbridge and Dorothy Anderson for all your hard work transcribing many interviews.

Eternal gratitude to Donna Canali, Mella Mincberg, and Moli Steinert for your continued support through the perpetual writing process.

Special thanks to my editor, Richard Leviton, and all the staff at Hampton Roads.

Contents

Introduction

We in the United States and other countries in the developed world are in the midst of a mental health crisis. The psychiatric treatment methods we have been using are not working, as is clear from the dire statistics on mental illness. Here are just a few:

- Mental illness is the second leading cause of disability and premature mortality in the U.S. and other developed countries.[1]

- 4 of the 10 leading causes of disability in the U.S. and other developed countries are mental disorders: schizophrenia, bipolar disorder, major depression, and obsessive-compulsive disorder.[2]

- 5.4 percent of adults in the U.S. have a serious mental illness (defined as "substantial interference with one or more major life activities"; less severe mental illness is not included in this statistic).[3]

- 1 in 4 hospital admissions in the U.S. in 1998 was a psychiatric admission.[4]

- In California alone, 20,000 to 30,000 people with mental illness are in prison; as many or more are homeless and live on the streets.[5]

- $148 billion = the cost of mental illness in the U.S. in a single year; $69 billion in direct costs for mental health treatment and rehabilitation and $79 billion in the indirect costs of lost productivity at work, school, or home due to disability or death.[6]

Largely, the reason that treatment of mental illness has a poor success record and is costing more all the time is that the overwhelming emphasis is placed on pharmaceutical drugs. Not everyone in the psychiatric field is happy with the ever-increasing governance of psychopharmacology (the science of drugs used to affect behavior and emotional states). Here is what one psychiatrist had to say about it. In December 1998, in a letter of resignation to the president of the American Psychiatric Association (APA), Loren R. Mosher, M.D., former official of the National Institute of Mental Health (NIMH), wrote:[7]

> After nearly three decades as a member, it is with a mixture of pleasure and disappointment that I submit this letter of resignation from the American Psychiatric Association. The major reason for this action is my belief that I am actually resigning from the American Psychopharmacological Association. . . . At this point in history, in my view, psychiatry has been almost completely bought out by the drug companies. . . . We condone and promote the widespread overuse and misuse of toxic chemicals that we know have serious long term effects. . . .

While psychiatric drugs (prescription drugs used for mental illnesses) may control certain disorders, and in some instances save lives, they do not cure the disorder, and they often compound the person's problems with disturbing side effects in the short term and the risk of permanent damage in the long term. If we are going to solve the current mental health crisis, we are going to have to turn to other approaches to treatment.

The state of affairs in psychiatric treatment is reflected in the focus of quite a few of the books on schizophrenia and other mental illness aimed at the general public. The help they offer involves information for the patient on coping with hospitalization; for family members on how to live with the illness in a loved one; and on how to work with side effects of psychopharmaceuticals (psychiatric drugs), that is, what other drugs you can take to reduce those effects.

Meanwhile, lives are sacrificed to schizophrenia, both literally and in the crippling of joy, potential, and quality of life that marks the illness unsuccessfully treated, as occurs far too often with the drug route. Even when drug treatment is considered "successful," most people face a lifetime on medication, and the underlying imbalances contributing to their condition are left unaddressed. People lose years of their lives as the illness ebbs and flows, despite their medications.

Are maintenance and endurance all we can hope for? The answer is no, despite conventional consensus to the contrary. *The Natural Medicine Guide to Schizophrenia* demonstrates that schizophrenia *is* treatable in many cases. The focus of the book is on healing from schizophrenia, not learning how to endure it. The case histories show that the use of natural approaches makes it possible for people to recover from schizophrenia and reclaim their lives. If implemented in mental hospitals and private practice, these therapies would revolutionize the psychiatric profession and change the very face of mental illness. If schizophrenia were not so devastating to the lives of those it touches, perhaps it would not be so vital that these therapies become part of standard protocol. As it is, where is the justification for not disseminating this information to all who are affected by schizophrenia?

The Natural Medicine Guide to Schizophrenia brings natural medicine treatment options together under one cover, so those with schizophrenia and their families can make informed choices about the treatment they pursue. The book explores the factors that can contribute to schizophrenia and offers a range of treatment approaches to address these factors and restore health on a deep level. Only by treating underlying imbalances, rather than suppressing the symptoms as most drugs do, can lasting recovery be achieved. And only by considering the well-being of the mind and spirit as well as the body can comprehensive healing take place.

The therapies covered in this book approach the treatment of schizophrenia in this way. They all also share the characteristic of tailoring treatment to the individual, which is another essential element for a successful outcome. No two people, even with the same diagnosis, have exactly the same imbalances causing their problems.

Natural therapies are those that operate according to holistic principles, meaning treating the whole person rather than an isolated part or symptom and using natural treatments that do no harm and support or restore the body's natural ability to heal itself. Natural medicine involves a way of looking at healing that is strikingly different from the conventional medical model. It does not mimic that model by merely substituting a nutritional supplement for a psychiatric drug. Instead, it is the comprehensive approach just described, which offers you the possibility of health.

Before I tell you a little about what's in the book, I have some comments about the terms "mental illness" and "mental disorders," or "brain disorders" as they are more currently labeled. All of these terms reflect the disconnection between body and mind—not to mention spirit—that characterizes conventional medical treatment. The newer term, brain disorders, reflects the biochemical model of causality that currently dominates the medical profession.

I use the terms "mental illness" and "mental disorders" in this book because there is no easy substitute that reflects the true body-mind-spirit nature of these conditions. While I may use these terms, I in no way mean to suggest that the causes of the disorders lie solely in the mind. The same is true for the title of the series of which this book is a part: The Healthy Mind Guides. The name serves to distinguish the subject area, but it is healthy mind, body, and spirit—wholeness—that is the focus of these books.

While I'm at it, I may as well dispense with one last linguistic issue. As natural medicine effects profound healing, rather than simply controlling symptoms, I prefer the term "natural medicine" over "alternative medicine." This medical model is not "other"—it is a primary form of medicine. The term "holistic medicine" reflects its primary nature as well, in that it signals the natural medicine approach of treating the whole person, rather than the parts.

Part 1 of *The Natural Medicine Guide to Schizophrenia* covers the basics of schizophrenia: what it is, who gets it, and what causes it. The natural medicine view is that it is a multicausal disorder, with a variety of contributing factors that need to be addressed in treatment.

Part 2 of the book covers a range of natural medicine treatments for schizophrenia. The material presented here is original information, not derivative material gleaned from secondary sources. It is based on interviews with physicians and other healing professionals who are leaders and pioneers in their respective fields.

For example, the doctors featured in the first two chapters—Abram Hoffer, M.D., Ph.D., and William J. Walsh, Ph.D.—are in the forefront of successful treatment of schizophrenia through nutritional protocols they have developed over decades of research. Their therapeutic approaches (orthomolecular medicine and biochemical therapy, respectively) have enabled thousands of people with schizophrenia to rejoin the community of people living full, productive lives. The case histories included in the chapters on their work are just a few of the many clinical successes made possible by the protocols developed by these brilliant doctors.

Among the other therapies covered in part 2 that have proven instrumental in ameliorating the symptoms of schizophrenia are anti-viral protocols, dental protocols, heavy metal detoxification, allergy elimination, cranial osteopathy to correct structural factors, constitutional homeopathy to restore energy balance, family systems therapy to clear transgenerational energy legacies, and psychosomatic medicine and shamanic healing to address psychospiritual factors.

This combination of therapies that cover the spectrum of body, mind, and spirit factors in schizophrenia is unique, as is the presentation. The methods of the highly skilled doctors and other healers included in this book are explained in detail and illustrated with case studies that give a human face to mental illness and demonstrate the effectiveness of the therapies. (The names of patients throughout the book have been changed.) Contact information for the practitioners whose work is presented appears in appendix B: Resources.

In the list of famous people with schizophrenia, which is found in chapter 1, you will find the name of Vaslav Nijinsky, to whom this book is dedicated. You may know the tragic story of this Russian dancer and choreographer (1890–1950), who is widely considered the greatest male dancer of the twentieth century. Not long after his ballet debut in St. Petersburg in 1907, he became the premier danseur in Diaghilev's Ballets Russes, a company that brought together the best musicians, painters, dancers, and choreographers of the time. Nijinsky danced his own choreography and that of others, defining roles in ballets that are still performed today. His rise was meteoric, as was his fall. In 1919, he left the world of dance forever, due to insanity, deemed in retrospect to be schizophrenia.

I dedicated this book to Nijinsky because for me he sums up the terrible loss of mental illness. The loss was brought home to me years ago when I saw Rudolf Nureyev dance a program of the ballets Nijinsky made famous, including his own *Afternoon of a Faun*. Nureyev, brilliant dancer that he was himself, seemed to have stepped aside to allow the spirit of Nijinsky to inhabit him and dance again. I sat in the top gallery of the theatre and wept, for Nijinsky and for all that he would have given the world had he not been felled by insanity.

This loss is shared by us all, just as is the loss of the contributions of each and every person, famous or otherwise, who is stopped by mental illness. It is my sincere hope that the information in this book helps you recover from schizophrenia, rejoin the dance of life, and give to the world the gifts you were meant to give.

Natural Medicine Therapies
Covered in Part II

Chap.	Health Practitioner	Therapies/Testing
3	Abram Hoffer, M.D., Ph.D. Michael Lesser, M.D. Hugh D. Riordan, M.D.	Orthomolecular medicine/psychiatry
4	William J. Walsh, Ph.D.	Biochemical therapy Urine and blood testing
5	Dietrich Klinghardt, M.D., Ph.D.	APN (applied psychoneuro-biology) Anti-viral protocol Chelation/heavy metal detoxification Family Systems Therapy NAET (allergy testing/elimination) Neural therapy
6	Lina Garcia, D.D.S., D.M.D.	Cranial osteopathy
7	Judyth Reichenberg-Ullman, N.D., L.C.S.W.	Constitutional homeopathy
8	Johannes Beckmann, M.D.	Psychosomatic medicine
9	Malidoma Patrice Somé, Ph.D.	Shamanic healing

1 What Is Schizophrenia, and Who Suffers from It?

Schizophrenia has long been a source of fascination, misunderstanding, mystery, and misery. Historically, it has been the most devastating of mental disorders in the degree of disability that it inflicts on those who suffer from it. It is to be hoped that this book will aid in both dispelling some of the misunderstandings and mystery around schizophrenia and changing the dismal prognosis that has heretofore been the lot of many who are diagnosed with the disease, despite the much-heralded antipsychotic drugs.

The National Institute of Mental Health describes schizophrenia as a "chronic, severe, and disabling brain disease," the seriousness of which is reflected in the epithet accorded schizophrenia in the psychiatric field: "the cancer of the mind."[8] Actually, schizophrenia is not a distinct disease, but a group of symptoms that show wide variation, characterized in general by disordered thinking, feelings, and behavior. A standard medical dictionary states that "there may be a precise disease called schizophrenia, but at this time, it is virtually impossible to distinguish it from a disease that may only resemble schizophrenia."[9]

No wonder misunderstanding reigns. The confusion is compounded by the widely held misconception that schizophrenia is a split personality, as in Robert Louis Stevenson's Dr. Jekyll and Mr. Hyde dichotomy, or even a multiple personality, as in the film

3

The Three Faces of Eve. This belief is perpetuated by the ubiquitous misuse of the word "schizophrenic," which has permeated our popular culture and is used to refer to a divide between opposites, à la Jekyll and Hyde, as in "schizophrenic management."

The misunderstanding stems in part from the roots of the word "schizophrenia," which was coined in 1908 by Swiss psychiatrist Eugen Bleuler and means "splitting of the mind."[10] Dr. Bleuler was referring to the disruption in thinking and feeling that accompanies the disorder, but the original meaning has gotten lost in common usage.

So, confusion reigns in both public and psychiatric spheres as to what exactly schizophrenia is. A summation of the confusion surrounding schizophrenia in medical circles notes that "schizophrenia has resisted definition to an even greater extent than it has resisted treatment."[11] In the absence of a distinct disease and laboratory findings such as brain abnormalities or other measurable physical anomalies, a diagnosis of schizophrenia depends upon symptomology.

 For more about imbalances and the levels of healing, see chapter 5.

The Symptoms of Schizophrenia

The symptoms of schizophrenia are generally divided into the categories of positive and negative symptoms, which is not a value judgment but a reflection of the deviation from normal function. Thus, positive symptoms are an excess or a distortion of normal functions, while negative symptoms are a lessening or a loss of normal functions.

Positive symptoms include delusions, hallucinations, paranoia, disorganized thinking and speaking, and disorganized or catatonic behavior. Negative symptoms include the "A" list: affective flattening (lack of emotional expression), avolition (lack of energy or initiative), alogia ("poverty of speech"), anhedonia (lack of pleasure or interest in previously enjoyable pursuits), and

Statistics on Schizophrenia

- 1 percent of the world population (1 to 2 out of 100 people in the U.S.) develops schizophrenia.

- More hospital beds in the U.S. are occupied by schizophrenic patients than by patients with any other illness, including cancer, heart disease, and stroke combined.

- Schizophrenia affects women and men nearly equally, with slightly more men being afflicted, but the onset tends to be earlier and the prognosis less positive among men.

- Schizophrenic onset generally occurs between the late teens and mid-thirties; the median age for men is the early to mid-twenties, while for women it is the late twenties.

- Children of two parents with schizophrenia have almost a 40 percent chance of becoming schizophrenic.

- 10 percent of schizophrenics commit suicide; up to 40 percent attempt suicide at least once.

- Schizophrenia in the U.S. costs $1 to 2 million per individual over a lifetime.

- The annual cost of schizophrenia is $48 billion (medical treatment, Social Security payments, and wages lost due to illness).

- Fewer than 50 percent of people with schizophrenia receive adequate treatment.[12]

In Their Own Words

"I recognized nothing, nobody. It was as though reality, attenuated, had slipped away from all these things and these people. Profound dread overwhelmed me, and as though lost, I looked around desperately for help. I heard people talking but I did not grasp the meaning of the words."[13]
—Renée, a recovered schizophrenic, co-author of *Autobiography of a Schizophrenic Girl*

attention deficits (concentration problems).

Loss of contact with reality is a hallmark of schizophrenia and the source of its categorization as a psychotic disorder. A sense of unreality, disconnection from the world, delusions, and hallucinations are all aspects of a distorted perception of reality. As with schizophrenia, the definition of psychosis is based upon symptoms, largely delusions and hallucinations.

Delusions are false beliefs or thoughts, while hallucinations are false sensory perceptions. The most common delusions involve persecution, as in the belief that you are being followed or watched or that people are talking about and ridiculing you. Other delusions focus on thought withdrawal, the belief that someone or something is taking away your thoughts; thought insertion, the belief that someone or something is putting thoughts into your head; or thought broadcasting, the belief that your thoughts are being transmitted to the world outside your head, often via radio or television. Religious delusions are also common, as in believing that one is Jesus or the Virgin Mary, or a less grandiose delusion.

Hallucinations can involve any of the senses. For example, a typical tactile hallucination among schizophrenics is the sensation of someone brushing against them as if in walking by, or nudging them, and there is nobody there. The most common hallucinations, however, are auditory, in which they hear voices, often conversations or someone issuing directives regarding their behavior.

In one instance, a woman with schizophrenia was forbidden by the voice in her head to eat anything but apples and spinach, and she knew from past experience with this voice that failure to observe the order would have dire consequences. The people around her naturally did not understand her dietary restrictions, but she had a very good reason for them.[14]

Her revelation raises an important point regarding logic, a word not often associated with madness. A number of the practitioners featured in this book emphasized that when they took the time to talk to their patients with schizophrenia, they discovered that they had logical reasons for why they behaved as they did. These logical reasons may have been based on delusions and hallucinations, but the point is that the seemingly bizarre behaviors were not random and had a kind of order of their own.

Another symptom that is often characteristic of schizophrenia, but which is not part of the official psychiatric symptom picture because it is subjective in nature rather than objectively observable, is a lack of awareness of physical boundaries. Not being clear on where one's body ends and people or objects in the outside world begin may be a function of sensory disturbance and an inability to process stimuli. Without this basic awareness, the person cannot have a strong sense of self. (See chapter 6 for another view of this phenomenon.)

Loss of contact with reality is linked to lack of insight, another feature in schizophrenia. The term refers to lack of awareness that one is ill, which makes the person less likely to be compliant with treatment. Research has found that this symptom is associated with a higher incidence of relapse, more involuntary hospitalizations, greater psychosocial impairment, and a poorer prognosis.[15]

Another hallmark of schizophrenia is disordered thinking. Thoughts (and speech, as an expression of thought) jump around, concentration and focus are difficult or nonexistent, mental associations are disrupted, and answers to questions posed to the individual may bear little or no perceivable relationship to the question. At its extreme manifestation, speech becomes what is known as "word salad," a jumble of words that seem incoherent to listeners.

"Grossly disorganized behavior," as it is termed in psychiatry, may include neglect of daily tasks such as making meals and bathing, dressing in an unusual manner (such as winter gear on a hot day), and having agitated outbursts (as in yelling or swearing), seemingly for no reason.

In Their Own Words

"If I do something, like going for a drink of water, I have to go over each detail. Find cup, walk over, turn tap, fill cup, turn tap off, drink it. I keep building up a picture. I have to change the picture each time. I have to make the old picture move. I can't concentrate. I can't hold things. . . . It's easier if I stay still."[16]

—A person with schizophrenia describing the loss of automatic movement

Of the negative symptoms of schizophrenia, flattened affect is quite often a feature. In this, the person has a blank look to observers and the face appears to be void of emotions or expression most of the time. Body language is similarly absent or reduced, as is eye contact. Another common negative symptom is alogia, in which the person answers or interacts with "brief, laconic, empty replies."[17]

Another way of characterizing the disorder, which summarizes the condition behind the symptoms, is that people with schizophrenia have trouble processing or filtering stimuli. E. Fuller Torrey, M.D., a clinical and research psychiatrist who specializes in schizophrenia, likens it to a switchboard operator failing to do the job of sorting and directing the incoming calls. Without this function, appropriate response becomes next to impossible. The limbic system of the brain acts as a filter (the switchboard) for sensory information; scientists suspect that this is the area most implicated in schizophrenia.[18]

The onset of schizophrenia, with some combination of the symptoms just cited, can be sudden or gradual, but there are usually signs that develop before the psychotic episode. These warning signs are clinically termed "prodromes" of the disease and include withdrawal from people and activities, lack of attention to appearance and cleanliness, and angry outbursts or other atypical behavior.

In addition to the symptoms associated with schizophrenia, there is a comorbidity factor with nicotine dependence, obsessive-compulsive disorder, and panic disorder.[19] Comorbidity means that two disorders exist together. Among people with schizophrenia, 80 to 90 percent are habitual cigarette smokers, and as such, nicotine dependent.[20] (See chapter 2 for more discussion of smoking and schizophrenia.)

Psychiatric Criteria for a Diagnosis of Schizophrenia

For a diagnosis of schizophrenia, according to the bible of the psychiatric profession, the *DSM-IV* (*Diagnostic and Statistical Manual of Mental Disorders, Fourth Edition*), at least two of the following symptoms must be present for "a significant portion of time" over a month (or less if treatment halts the symptoms):[21]

1. Delusions
2. Hallucinations
3. Disorganized speech
4. Grossly disorganized or catatonic behavior
5. Negative symptoms such as affective flattening, alogia, or avolition.

The presence of bizarre delusions or auditory hallucinations in which a voice makes continual comments about the individual or two or more people are heard in conversation obviates the requirement for two symptoms.

While these "active-phase" symptoms must last at least a month, there must be signs of disturbance for six months or more. These signs may be negative symptoms or less severe positive symptoms such as unusual perceptions or beliefs.

In addition, diagnosis requires that there is a marked decrease in the person's social, occupational, and/or self-care functioning since the disturbance began (or in the case of children, their functioning in these areas fails to develop as expected).

Finally, it must be determined that these symptoms are not due to other causes. That is, schizoaffective disorder (see following section), mood disorder, medical conditions, and substance-induced psychosis must be ruled out. This is because medical conditions such as Cushing's syndrome or a brain tumor can produce schizophrenia-like symptoms, as can street

> ## In Their Own Words
>
> *"When people are talking, I just get scraps of it. If it is just one person who is speaking, that's not so bad, but if others join in, then I can't pick it up at all."[22]*
> —A person with schizophrenia describing perceptual disruption

drugs, medications, or toxic exposure (see chapter 2).

Types of Schizophrenia

In addition to the main category of schizophrenia, there are a number of subtypes and alternative diagnostic labels, as defined in the *DSM-IV*. A holistic medical approach does not use such diagnoses to determine the appropriate treatment course, focusing instead on the particular manifestations and underlying imbalances in the individual patient. Nevertheless, as many people receive these labels, it's helpful to know to what they refer.

Schizophrenia Subtypes

A person may fit into more than one subtype, and two of them are vague categories for use when people don't fit anywhere else. Even the authors of the *DSM-IV* admit that due to the "limited value of the schizophrenia subtypes in clinical and research settings (e.g., prediction of course, treatment response, correlates of illness), alternative subtyping schemes are being actively investigated."[23] In other words, the diagnostic subtypes don't serve much purpose aside from, in the case of three of them, describing the primary symptoms.

Paranoid Type

Paranoid schizophrenia is characterized by delusions or auditory hallucinations, without significant impairment of thinking and feeling. The delusions involved are usually of the persecution and/or grandiose type. The hallucinations typically relate to the theme found in the delusions. Anxiety, anger, aloofness, and a tendency to argue are also common. The onset of paranoid schizophrenia is usually later than with other types and the prognosis is better because of mild to nonexistent disturbance in thinking.

Disorganized Type

As suggested by its name, the main characteristic of this type of schizophrenia is disorganization of speech and behavior. Flattened or inappropriate emotional expression (such as laughter with no apparent connection to speech content) is also present. If the person has hallucinations or delusions, they too tend to be disorganized, rather than relating to a theme as is the case with the paranoid type. The disorganization in behavior can result in major disturbance in daily activities. Early onset and lack of remission also characterize the disorganized type of schizophrenia.[24]

> ### In Their Own Words
>
> *"I thought I was telepathic. I thought everybody in the world had read my mind and that they had a negative impression of me. So when I thought that I had caused people in different provinces [in Canada] to commit suicide because of me blasting them with waves of telepathic neurotic hatred, I thought, 'Well, now they're going to get me.'"[25]*
> —Ian, who reversed his schizophrenia with orthomolecular medicine

Catatonic Type

Catatonia is characterized by psychomotor symptoms that range from immobility to excessive movement, from holding a fixed posture to stupor (a total lack of response to and seeming unawareness of one's environment). Grimacing, echolalia (repetition of others' words or phrases), and echopraxia (repetitive mimicking of others' movements) are also common.

Undifferentiated Type

According to the *DSM-IV,* the undifferentiated type meets the criteria for a diagnosis of schizophrenia, but does not fall into the paranoid, disorganized, or catatonic subtypes.

Residual Type

This type of schizophrenia may reflect the transition from a psychotic episode to remission, but can be operational for years.

To meet the criteria for the residual type, the person must have had at least one schizophrenic episode, but delusions, hallucinations, and other positive symptoms are at this time not significant. Negative symptoms are present, however.

Other Diagnostic Categories

The diagnostic labels schizophreniform disorder and schizoaffective disorder are used when the criteria for a diagnosis of schizophrenia are not met but the disorder shares a number of features with schizophrenia. The *DSM-IV* also cites other psychotic disorders, but it is sufficient for our purposes to limit discussion to these two.

Schizophreniform Disorder

For this diagnosis, the person meets the criteria for schizophrenia, except that the illness (prodromal, active, and residual stages) has lasted less than six months and there may or may not be disturbance in the person's social and professional function. If the illness meets all the criteria for schizophrenia except the duration and it then lasts past the six-month mark, the diagnosis will become schizophrenia.

Schizoaffective Disorder

While this disorder is listed under schizophrenia in the *DSM-IV,* it is defined as involving a major depressive, manic, or mixed episode (both mania and depression) in combination with two or more of the characteristic symptoms of schizophrenia: delusions, hallucinations, disorganized speech, catatonic or grossly disorganized behavior, or negative symptoms such as flat affect, alogia, or avolition. Schizoaffective disorder presents very much like bipolar disorder (the mood disorder formerly known as manic-depression) with psychotic features, the difference being that delusions and hallucinations in the latter case are part of the abnormal mood, while no such relationship exists in schizoaffective disorder.[26]

People with schizophrenia are frequently diagnosed with bipolar disorder and vice versa. Others receive a dual diagnosis of schizophrenia and bipolar disorder. The schizoaffective category highlights the confusion in attempting to distinguish between the disorders.

 For information about bipolar disorder, see the author's *The Natural Medicine Guide to Bipolar Disorder* (Hampton Roads, 2003).

The Demographics of Schizophrenia

Schizophrenia affects about one percent of the population worldwide, with some evidence suggesting that there are slight variations according to geography and culture. For example, research indicates that more people are afflicted in the northern hemisphere as compared to the southern, and the closer one is to the equator the less likely one is to develop schizophrenia.[27] In addition, Papua, New Guinea, has a very low rate while western Ireland, Sweden, and the Istrian peninsula in Croatia purportedly have very high rates. The incidence is also high among Caribbean immigrants in England (but not high in their native countries, with the exception perhaps of Dominica).[28] In the past 20 years, the incidence of schizophrenia has reportedly decreased in Scotland, England, Denmark, Australia, and New Zealand, while some evidence suggests that it has increased in the United States.[29] As with so much else about schizophrenia, the causes for these changes and variations are a mystery.

The type, course, and outcome of the illness vary across cultures as well, with catatonic schizophrenia more common in developing countries than in industrialized countries. Schizophrenia in the latter tends to be chronic and have a worse outcome while in the former it is usually acute and has a better prognosis.[30] One World Health Organization (WHO) study found that a large percentage of people with severe schizophrenia in less industrialized cultures where extended families are the norm recovered completely, unlike in the industrialized world, where nuclear families are the norm. Further, the WHO study found that the availability of psychiatric drug treatment is correlated with more negative outcomes for people with schizophrenia.[31]

Incidence rates are almost twice as high in urban, as opposed to rural, locations, with the poor in the cities most affected. Some research found a higher rate of schizophrenia among African Americans, but further investigation determined that this is due more to residence in cities than to race. Among rural-dwelling African Americans, the incidence is no higher than normal.[32]

The World Health Organization study found that the availability of psychiatric drug treatment is correlated with more negative outcomes for people with schizophrenia.

Schizophrenia tends to run in families and usually manifests in late adolescence or early adulthood. Fewer than one percent of people with schizophrenia have an onset before age 12, and fewer than ten percent have an onset after age 45.[33] The peak age of onset is the early to mid-twenties for men and the late twenties for women.[34] As with bipolar disorder, the average age of onset has dropped from what it was 20 years ago. Again, the reason is unknown.

Violence, Suicide, and Schizophrenia

A common myth about schizophrenia is that people with the disorder are violent. The myth is fueled by the occasional, highly publicized act of violence committed by a diagnosed schizophrenic, typically against a famous person. While there is disagreement over whether people with schizophrenia are more likely than nonschizophrenics to perpetrate violence against others, the official stance of the National Institute of Mental Health (NIMH) is: "Most individuals with schizophrenia are not violent; more typically, they are withdrawn and prefer to be left alone. Most violent crimes are not commited by persons with schizophrenia, and most persons with schizophrenia do not commit violent crimes."[35] There is evidence that the same factors that increase the likelihood of violence in the general population are those that increase the likelihood among people with schizophrenia. These include drug abuse, being young, male, and poor.[36]

When it comes to violence against self, however, schizophrenics are more likely than the general population to harm themselves, with the ultimate harm being suicide. As many as 40 percent of people with schizophrenia attempt suicide at least once, while ten percent of schizophrenics succeed in killing themselves.[37] Alcohol abuse increases the likelihood of suicide, as alcohol features in 30 percent of all suicides.[38]

The high incidence of suicide attempts among people with schizophrenia makes it important for those with the condition, as well as their family and friends, to be aware of the warning signs of suicide. Being forewarned may enable you to prevent this tragedy from happening if the signs begin to manifest. Among schizophrenics, increased risk factors include being male, under 45 years old, unemployed, depressed or hopeless, and recently discharged from the hospital.[39] In general, the warning signs of suicide are[40]

- feelings of hopelessness, worthlessness, anguish, or desperation
- withdrawal from people and activities
- preoccupation with death or morbid subjects
- sudden mood improvement or increased activity after a period of depression
- increase in risk-taking behaviors
- buying a gun
- putting affairs in order
- thinking, talking, or writing about a plan for committing suicide

If you think that you or someone you know is in danger of attempting suicide, call your doctor or a suicide hotline or get

Factors Associated with a Better Outcome

Research has linked the following factors to a more positive prognosis in schizophrenia.[41]

Good adjustment prior to
    becoming ill
Acute onset
Onset at a later age
Being a female
Accompanying mood
    disturbance
Treatment soon after onset
Good functioning between
    episodes
Minimal residual symptoms
No structural brain
    abnormalities
Normal functioning of the
    nervous system
Awareness of illness
Family history of mood
    disorders
No family history of
    schizophrenia

help from another qualified source. Know that there is help and, though it may be difficult to ask for it, a life may depend upon it.

Schizophrenia and Creativity

There is another side to schizophrenia, and that is its possible link to creativity. Madness in general has long been paired with genius in the arts. Investigation reveals that there is some substance behind what some dismiss as a romantic notion.

Psychiatrist E. Fuller Torrey, M.D., cites the cognitive traits that characterize creative people and people with schizophrenia: "Both use words and language in unusual ways (the hallmark of a great poet or novelist), both have unusual views of reality (as great artists do), both often utilize unusual thought processes in their deliberations, and both tend to prefer solitude to the company of others."[42]

In addition, Dr. Torrey reports that psychological testing of creative people reveals more "psychopathology" as compared to noncreative people. At the same time, nonparanoid schizophrenics test very high on creativity tests. Another study found that the immediate family members of a creative person appear to be more likely to develop schizophrenia, and similarly, the immediate family members of a schizophrenic person test higher for creativity.[43]

The connection between madness and creativity is not fully understood. Does the artistic process promote madness or are people suffering from mental illness temperamentally drawn to the arts? Whatever the answer, it is important not to lose sight of the tragic aspect of the madness-genius equation, which can get lost in the romanticization of the artistic life. As Kay Redfield Jamison, Ph.D., author of *Touched with Fire*, an exploration of the connection between madness and creativity, observes, "No one is creative when paralytically depressed, psychotic, institutionalized, in restraints, or dead because of suicide."[44]

Famous People with Schizophrenia

The following are among the well-known people who suffered from schizophrenia:[45]

Antonin Artaud, writer
Ivor Gurney, poet/composer
Jakob Adolf Hagg, composer
Johann Friedrich Hölderlin, poet
John Forbes Nash, Jr., Nobel prize-winning mathematician (the subject of the film *A Beautiful Mind*)
Vaslav Nijinsky, dancer/choreographer
Adolf Wolfli, painter

Possibly:

James Joyce, writer
August Strindberg, writer
Vincent van Gogh, painter

The History of Schizophrenia and Its Treatment

In the history of schizophrenia is also found the muddied confusion that surrounds other aspects of the disorder. While some authorities maintain that schizophrenia has afflicted humans throughout time, others aver that it is a relatively modern disorder that came into existence in the early 1800s.

Proponents of the age-old view cite a description of what they believe to be schizophrenia found in Hindu scriptures dating from around 1400 B.C. Seen as the victim of devils, the person "is gluttonous, is filthy, walks naked, has lost his memory, and moves about in an uneasy manner."[46] Biblical descriptions of insanity are considered further support for this position.

Those who believe that schizophrenia is a more recent phenomenon acknowledge that psychoses resembling schizophrenia may have existed but that the causes were disease or injury and not the entity we know as schizophrenia. While isolated descriptions of schizophrenia-like conditions appeared in the seventeenth and eighteenth centuries, there was a sudden flood of descriptions in the nineteenth century, beginning with what proponents of this view cite as the first definite descriptions of schizophrenia. These were published independently in 1809 by both English physician John Haslam and French physician Philippe Pinel.

One school of thought maintains that the flood of descriptions was a reflection of a huge increase in mental illness in Europe during the 1800s. Various arguments, such as the advent of industrialization leading to workers no longer taking care of insane family members in the home, attempt to explain away this phenomenon, but analysis by some authorities has resulted in the conclusion that the increase did indeed occur. A huge increase in madness purportedly occurred in the United States as well, as reflected in a dramatic rise in the number of mental hospitals. Again, the reason for the increase, if such it was, is not known.

Whether schizophrenia existed as a distinct disorder before the 1800s or not, people who were deemed insane were subjected to a range of "medical" treatments over the years. In the view of the ancient world and later in the Middle Ages, the insane were regarded as victims of demon possession and, as such, needed to be treated with compassion. Torture and persecution of the insane commenced with the witch-burnings, beginning in the fifteenth century, and continued through the 1700s.

In the 1800s, the cause of schizophrenia was considered unknown, although environment, heredity, and organic disease were variously proposed as the source of the ailment. Hospital reform during this era led to more humane treatment of the insane. The methods for treating schizophrenia that evolved in the nineteenth and twentieth centuries included immersion in hot or cold baths, inducing fevers, inducing an insulin coma, and electroconvulsive therapy (shock treatment).

The year 1852 brought the introduction of the term *dementia praecox,* the early name for schizophrenia. Benedict Morel dubbed the illness he was witnessing in the French mental institute where he served as the head physician *démence précoce* (early or premature loss of mind), referring to its early onset. The clinical version of this is the Latin *dementia praecox.* As noted earlier, it wasn't until the the early 1900s that the term "schizophrenia" came into usage.

In the late 1800s, German physician Emil Kraepelin studied and documented schizophrenia and other mental illnesses, providing the foundation for modern psychiatry. Its focus on diagnosis and classification comes from Dr. Kraepelin.[47]

The belief that psychological factors were the cause of mental illnesses arose from the work of Sigmund Freud and began to gain cachet in the American medical establishment in the 1920s.[48] With the source of such illness firmly placed in the mind, parents (mostly mothers), early trauma, and psychological conflicts became the culprits behind schizophrenia, bipolar disorder, and autism. This orientation is largely responsible for the stigma that came to be attached to mental illness—that is, that schizophrenia is not a disease like any other, but a failing on the part of the individual or the individual's mother.

The so-called schizophrenogenic mother (a woman whose maladjusted mothering caused her child's schizophrenia) or the "frozen mother" (whose withholding of love caused the schizophrenia in her child) are close relatives of the "refrigerator mother" whose lack of emotional engagement was blamed for autism. Before the psychological model gave way to the biochemical model of mental illness, these labels caused further anguish in families already dealing with the painful realities of having a schizophrenic child.

The advent of psychiatric drugs in the 1950s transformed the psychiatric field, shifting the focus of the causality of mental illness to the biochemical realm and turning the profession into a pharmaceutical industry. Gradually, the medical redefinition with its focus on biology permeated public consciousness, but the stigma attached to mental illness persists to a certain degree. This is especially true of schizophrenia, which has not reaped the benefits that other mental disorders have from celebrities going public about their bipolar disorder or clinical depression and helping to dispel some of the earlier judgments and misconceptions. Medically, the role of psychological factors in schizophrenia is dismissed or considered minimal and the focus of treatment is on drugs.

In the United States, another development in the mental health field had serious consequences that are still reverberating through society and among the mentally ill today. A policy of deinstitutionalization, initiated across the country in the late 1960s, resulted in massive closure of state and county mental hospitals. From 1969 to 1975 alone, the schizophrenic population in such facilities dropped by nearly half.[49] These people were now supposed to receive treatment on an outpatient basis, but services were woefully inadequate. The result has been catastrophic. Nationwide, "90 percent of the people who would have been in the hospital 40 years ago are not in the hospital today," states Dr. Torrey.[50]

In California, where the 1967 Lanterman Petris Short (LPS) Act led to the closure of many mental hospitals and the abolishment of staff positions in many others, the state mental hospital population dropped from 35,739 in 1968 (the year before LPS took effect) to 4,000 in 1999. "Between 20,000 and 30,000 people with mental illness are in our jails and prisons. At least an equal number are homeless on the street," reads a report by a task force that investigated the impact of this law in California.[51] This tragic situation exists throughout the United States.

"The new mental hospitals are the streets," observes Abram Hoffer, M.D., Ph.D., whose work with schizophrenia is covered in chapter 3.[52]

An estimated one-third of those who are homeless suffer from severe mental illness, predominantly schizophrenia.

One could add that jails and prisons are also our new mental hospitals. "It is easier for a person with a severe mental illness to get arrested than to get treatment," reads a statement in a report by the National Alliance for the Mentally Ill (NAMI). The report cites the lack of community services for the mentally ill as the cause of "the growing criminalization of persons with severe mental illnesses." According to NAMI statistics, more than 10 percent of jail and prison inmates suffer from schizophrenia, bipolar disorder, or major depression.[53]

The criminalization of the mentally ill carries with it the issue of forced medication. The incarcerated mentally ill have been forcibly medicated, and court cases either challenging the practice or seeking to continue it have arisen.[54] Without federal guidelines on the issue, it continues to be heard on a case-by-case basis. Meanwhile, many inmates are forced against their will to take powerful antipsychotics. This has serious implications for those who wish to follow an alternative route of treatment, such as the therapeutic approaches enumerated in this book.

> ## In Their Own Words
>
> "Robert's diagnosis has changed frequently in the past 30 years, depending largely upon which drugs have been successful in keeping him calm, stable, and/or compliant. He was schizophrenic when enormous doses of Thorazine and Stelazine calmed him; he was manic-depressive (bipolar) when lithium worked; he was manic-depressive-with-psychotic-symptoms, or hypomanic, when Tegretol or Depakote (anticonvulsants), or some new antipsychotic or antidepressant . . . showed promise of making him cooperative. . . ."[55]
>
> —Jay Neugeboren, about his brother Robert's illness

The Pharmacological Age

Antipsychotic medications now rule conventional psychiatric treatment of schizophrenia. The current conventional view is that schizophrenia is a brain disorder involving some kind of neurotransmitter malfunction, so drugs thought to manipulate neurotransmitter function are the prescribed course of treatment.

Neurotransmitters are the brain's chemical messengers that enable communication between cells. While there are many different kinds of neurotransmitters, the primary ones thought to be involved in schizophrenia are dopamine, serotonin, epineph-rine/norepinephrine, GABA (gamma-aminobutyric acid), and glutamate.

Much of the research on neurotransmitters and schizophrenia has focused on dopamine, largely because Thorazine, an antipsy-chotic drug that reduced the symptoms of schizophrenia and was the standard treatment until other antipsychotics were developed, was found to reduce dopamine activity. In fact, this drug-spurred approach has been the basis for much of the neurotransmitter research. Serotonin got attention because clozapine, another antipsychotic drug used with schizophrenia, affected serotonin.

One theory holds that dopamine may be operating to excess in severe mania and acute schizophrenia,[56] but recent research sug-gests that this is too simplistic given the complexity of the dopamine system.[57] Dopamine has a role in memory retrieval, attention, mood regulation, and the processing of experience, emotion, and thought.[58]

Serotonin influences mood, regulates sleep and pain, and is involved in sensory perception, all of which have relevance to schizophrenia. Contrary to popular belief, serotonin is not found only in the brain. In fact, only five percent of the body's supply is in the brain, with 95 percent distributed throughout the body and involved in many functions.[59] Serotonin is similarly distrib-uted throughout the brain, where it is "the single largest brain sys-tem known."[60]

Epinephrine (also known as adrenaline) and norepineph-rine are hormones produced by the adrenal gland. Epinephrine is involved in the stress response and the physiology of fear and anxiety; an excess has been implicated in some anxiety disorders. Norepinephrine is similar to epinephrine and is the form of adrenaline found in the brain.[61] It plays a role in cognitive func-tions such as attention, learning, and mental sharpness. Interference with norepinephrine metabolism at certain brain sites has been linked to affective disorders.[62] Paranoia, aggres-sion, and anger may result from high levels; note that ampheta-mines, which raise norepinephrine levels, can produce similar effects.[63]

Prescription Drugs Used to Control Schizophrenia

Antipsychotics (typical)
haloperidol (Haldol)
thioridazine (Mellaril)
fluphenazine (Prolixin)
trifluoperazine (Stelazine)
chlorpromazine (Thorazine)

Antipsychotics (atypical)
clozapine (Clozaril)
risperidone (Risperdal)
quetiapine (Seroquel)
olanzapine (Zyprexa)

Anticholinergics
   Also called antiparkinsonian or side-effect medication; used to counteract the side effects of antipsychotics
trihexyphenidyl (Artane)
benztropine mesylate
   (Cogentin)
procyclidine (Kemadrin)
amantadine (Symmetrel)

Antidepressants
trazodone (Desyrel)

paroxetine (Paxil)
fluoxetine (Prozac)
sertraline (Zoloft)

Mood stabilizers
valproic acid (Depakene)
divalproex (Depakote)
lamotrigine (Lamictal)
lithium carbonate
carbamazepine (Tegretol), an
   anticonvulsant
topiramate (Topamax)

Tranquilizers
   Benzodiazepines, anxiolytics (anti-anxiety medications)
lorazepam (Ativan)
clonazepam (Klonopin)
diazepam (Valium)
alprazolam (Xanax)

Anti-Panic Drugs
clonazepam (Klonopin)
paroxetine (Paxil)
alprazolam (Xanax)
sertraline (Zoloft)

GABA operates to stop excess nerve stimulation, thereby exerting a calming effect on the brain. GABA is involved in 30 to 50 percent of brain synapses (the juncture between two nerve cells on the pathways along which communications in the brain travel).[64] Two important functions of glutamate involve memory and the curbing of chronic stress response and excess secretion of the adrenal "stress" hormone cortisol. Stimulus adaptation, which is impaired in schizophrenia, is thus the purview of glutamate.[65]

Neurotransmitters are ostensibly the targets of psychiatric drugs used in the treatment of mental illness, although it is unknown exactly how these drugs work. In the case of schizophrenia, these drugs fall into the categories of antipsychotics (typical and atypical), mood stabilizers, antidepressants, and tranquilizers. While the effects and side effects of all could be enumerated at length, the following brief discussion focuses on antipsychotics, which are the mainstay of drug prescription for schizophrenia.

Antipsychotics, also known as neuroleptics (the literal translation is "taking hold of the nerves"), and formerly referred to as major tranquilizers, work to control schizophrenia by blunting a range of brain activities. They produce "apathy, indifference, emotional blandness, conformity, and submissiveness, as well as a reduction in all verbalizations, including complaints or protests," according to Peter R. Breggin, M.D., and David Cohen, Ph.D., authors of *Your Drug May Be Your Problem.* "It is no exaggeration to call this effect a chemical lobotomy."[66] The phrase "the Thorazine shuffle" came into usage in mental hospitals in the early days of Thorazine prescription, referring to the characteristic way of moving as a result of the numbing physical, mental, and emotional effects of this primary neuroleptic.

Although antipsychotics are ostensibly given to control delusions and hallucinations, they actually have no specific effects on either, say Drs. Breggin and Cohen, and their side effects are daunting. In addition to those cited, side effects of this class of drugs include dry mouth, blurred vision, drowsiness, restlessness, muscle spasms, and tremors. They can also cause side effects that resemble psychotic symptoms.[67]

A serious long-term effect of neuroleptic drugs is tardive dyskinesia (TD), characterized by involuntary muscle movement, most often afflicting the limbs, mouth, tongue, eyes, and other parts of the face. Involuntary grimaces, tongue protusions, lip smacking, and chewing are typical manifestations. TD can be a permanent disability, meaning that it persists even when the drug is discontinued. TD indicates that the drug has damaged the brain in some way, but the medical profession tends to downplay the problem.

In a pamphlet written by a team of psychiatrists at the Clarke Institute of Psychiatry in the Department of Psychiatry at the University of Toronto to provide information to patients and their families on medications for schizophrenia, the authors state the following in regard to TD: "[T]he benefits of medication must be weighed against the adverse effects, and most people who have tardive dyskinesia are less disturbed by it than are their relatives and friends. In other words, the effects are unsightly but not necessarily uncomfortable."[68] Might the presence of this misleading and presumptuous, even outrageous, statement have anything to do with an illuminating note at the end of the pamphlet? "This booklet has been provided by The Professional Services Department of Merrell Dow Pharmaceuticals (Canada) Inc."[69]

While the risks associated with neuroleptics are considered by many to be worth it if the drug can control an adult's schizophrenia, there can be no justification for the growing use of antipsychotics on children for whom the drugs are not approved and for whom the purpose has nothing to do with schizophrenia.

While so-called atypical antipsychotics, such as Zyprexa, are enjoying cachet now over Thorazine and other typical antipsychotics because their side effects are regarded as less onerous, Drs. Breggin and Cohen strongly state: "All neuroleptics produce an enormous variety of potentially severe and disabling neurological impairments at extraordinarily high rates of occurrence; they are among the most toxic agents ever administered to people."[70]

Bernard Rimland, Ph.D., director of the Autism Research Institute in San Diego, California, coined the term "toximolecular" in reference to the psychiatric practice of treating mental illnesses with "sublethal doses of substances that will kill you."[71]

Toximolecular medicine is in direct contrast to orthomolecular medicine, which is the use of natural substances to bring about health (see chapter 3).

While the risks associated with neuroleptics are considered by many to be worth it if the drug can control an adult's schizophrenia, there can be no justification for the growing use of antipsychotics on children for whom the drugs are not approved and for whom the purpose has nothing to do with schizophrenia (see sidebar). It should also be noted that 30 to 60 percent of people with schizophrenia are drug-resistant to neuroleptics, which means the drugs don't work.[72]

Atypical antipsychotics are supposed to be less likely to produce TD than the older, typical antipsychotics, but there is still a risk. More common side effects of the newer class of drugs include dizziness, drowsiness, drooling, weight gain, fatigue, dry mouth, lowered blood pressure, rapid heart beat, constipation, social withdrawal, and Parkinsonian-like symptoms.[73]

In the case of clozapine, it can cause a condition known as agranulocytosis, a potentially fatal disease in which the manufacture of white blood cells is dangerously curtailed.[74] Clozapine and risperidone can produce neuroleptic malignant syndrome, another potentially fatal disease, this one of the brain, with symptoms similar to those of viral encephalitis.[75] And these drugs are considered less onerous than the typical antipsychotics!

As with typical antipsychotics, science does not know exactly how atypical antipsychotics work. One research team summarized, "The precise pharmacologic mechanisms underlying 'atypicality' remain unclear. . . ."[76] Further, although the new drugs are touted as an improvement over the old in effectiveness and reduced side effects, research calls this claim into question. One study analyzed 52 randomized trials, with a total of 12,649 subjects with schizophrenia, and concluded, "There is no clear evidence that atypical antipsychotics are more effective or are better tolerated than conventional antipsychotics."[77] One feature strongly differentiates the new class of drugs from the old, however: they are far more expensive. So much so that some people's medical coverage won't pay for them.

When side effects are disturbing, more drugs are prescribed to counteract them. These drugs are known as anticholinergic (blocking certain nerve impulses), antiparkinsonian (Parkinson's

More Children Are Getting Antipsychotic Drugs

A new and disturbing trend in conventional medicine and psychiatry is the increasing use of antipsychotic medications to control children's behavior. About 532,000 children, between the ages of six and 18, are on these drugs. This number comprises only non-hospitalized children, not those who are on the drugs as part of inpatient treatment. The number is more than ten times what it was ten years ago, and back then most children receiving antipsychotics were in a treatment facility of some kind.

Atypical antipsychotics such as Risperdal and Zyprexa are being prescribed to children, not because they have been diagnosed with childhood schizophrenia, but to curb aggressive behavior such as hitting and biting. While the FDA has approved these drugs for use in treating adult schizophrenia, it has not approved their use in children, much less as a treatment for aggression. Doctors, however, can legally prescribe them to children on what is known as an "off-label" basis, which means that the drug is being used outside of approval parameters.

Research on the use of atypical antipsychotics in children is appallingly inadequate: study of the effects of these drugs amounts to looking at approximately 500 children for one year. Neither the short-term nor the long-term effects of these drugs on developing bodies is known.[78]

A growing number of children are also being put on antidepressants, despite the fact that Prozac and similar antidepressants are approved by the FDA only for use in patients over the age of 18.[79] There has been very little research, even on adults, on the long-term effects of taking antidepressants such as Prozac. It is known, however, that this class of antidepressants can produce neurological disorders, and permanent brain damage is a danger.[80]

Add to this the alarming number of children who have been diagnosed with ADD/ADHD (attention deficit/hyperactivity disorder) and are on drugs such as Ritalin, and it could be said that the youth of today are entering adulthood heavily medicated. The implications of this have yet to be revealed.

disease is characterized by tremors and an odd gait), or side-effect medications. They produce side effects of their own, ranging from blurred vision to severe psychiatric symptoms such as hallucinations, delusions, and paranoia, and an increased risk of tardive dyskinesia. Some doctors maintain that when anticholinergics are used on a long-term basis, "irreversible mental deterioration" can result.[81]

In addition to antipsychotics and side-effect medication, mood stabilizers, antidepressants, tranquilizers, and/or anti-panic medications may be added to the schizophrenic's drug "cocktail." Most people with schizophrenia face a lifetime on these drugs because they are not a cure, but only a means of controlling the symptoms, and often not well at that.

There is no doubt that antipsychotic and other drugs save lives. The purpose of the previous discussion is not to advocate the elimination of these drugs, but to point out their dangers and the advisability of finding an alternative where possible. The latter is indicated, not only because of the negative effects of psychiatric medications, but also because the pharmacological model is basically flawed. Drugs do not address the underlying factors that cause or contribute to the condition. With drug-based treatment, these factors go uninvestigated and the best one can hope for is maintenance.

Natural medicine, on the other hand, is based on the knowledge that in order for comprehensive healing to occur, the factors causing or contributing to a disorder must be identified and addressed in each person. With this approach, it is possible for people with schizophrenia to get off their psychiatric drugs or significantly reduce their dosages and improve their present and future health. The next chapter explores the underlying factors that can play a role in schizophrenia.

2 Causes, Triggers, and Contributors

The cause of schizophrenia is unknown, but the current medical view is that environmental factors of some kind combine with a genetic vulnerability to trigger the disorder. The reality is that, in spite of widespread acceptance in the medical community, the disease model of schizophrenia, the genetic component, and the focus on neurotransmitter dysfunction as the source of the problem are all suspect.

Here is what some eminent psychiatrists and researchers say on the subject:

> [T]here is no proven physical cause for any psychiatric disorder. . . . [W]hy are so many . . . convinced that the origins of mental illnesses are to be found in biology, when, despite more than three decades of research, there is still no proof? . . . The absence of any well-defined physical causation is reflected in the absence of any laboratory tests for psychiatric diagnoses—much in contrast to diabetes and many other physical disorders.
>
> —Charles E. Dean, M.D., director of psychiatric residency at the Minneapolis Veterans Medical Center, quoted in the *Minnesota Star Tribune* (November 22, 1997).[82]

Contrary to what is often claimed, no biochemical, anatomical or functional signs have been found that reliably distinguish the brains of mental patients.

—Dr. Elliot Valenstein, Ph.D., University of Michigan neuroscientist and professor emeritus of psychology, author of *Blaming the Brain: The Truth About Drugs and Mental Health.*[83]

[W]e have no identified etiological agents for psychiatric disorders.

—Gary J. Tucker, M.D., professor and chairman of psychiatry and behavioral sciences at the University of Washington School of Medicine, quoted in the *American Journal of Psychiatry* (February 1998).[84]

Through the 1970s and 1980s, a curious circularity invaded psychiatry, as "diseases" began to be "modeled" on the medications that "treat" them. If a drug elevated serotonin in test tubes, then it was presumptuously argued that patients helped by the medication must have serotonin deficiencies even though we lack scientific proof for the idea.

—Joseph Glenmullen, M.D., clinical instructor in psychiatry at Harvard Medical School and author of *Prozac Backlash.*[85]

From a holistic viewpoint, a physiological cause alone or in combination with a genetic abnormality, is not the sum total of a condition such as schizophrenia. Perhaps research has been unable to identify an "etiological agent" because "mental illness" is the outcome of body-mind-spirit disturbance caused by physical, psychological, emotional, spiritual, and energetic influences, each of which affects all of the other areas so no influence can be considered in isolation.

If we acknowledge that body, mind, and spirit cannot be separated (conventional medicine acknowledges at least the first two; even the surgeon general of the United States has stated that mind and body are "inseparable"[86]), then we should not look only to one area for the cause and the solution. Even if the source arises in one area, the reverberations, like ripples in a pond, extend throughout the body, mind, and spirit and are soon indistinguishable as cause or effect.

To recover from schizophrenia, it is not necessary to know the exact causal mechanism, but it is necessary to identify and treat the existing imbalances in each individual case. The approach must be individualized because the combination of factors differs and the specifics of each factor vary from person to person.

With that in mind, this chapter looks at 21 factors that can contribute to, trigger, exacerbate, or mimic schizophrenia. While a particular factor may seem to be predominantly physical, psychological, or spiritual in nature, remember the ripple-in-the-pond effect and know that it will have an effect on the other areas as well.

1. Familial Vulnerability

"No claim of a gene for a psychiatric condition has stood the test of time, in spite of popular misinformation,"

21 Factors in Schizophrenia

The following can exacerbate, trigger, contribute to, or mimic schizophrenia:

familial vulnerability

stress

chemical toxicity

heavy metal toxicity

food allergies

intestinal dysbiosis

sensitivity to food additives

nutritional deficiencies/ imbalances

neurotransmitter deficiencies or dysfunction

structural factors

viruses

hypoglycemia

hormonal imbalances

medical conditions

medications

street drugs

caffeine, alcohol, and nicotine

lack of sleep

lack of exercise

energy imbalances

psychospiritual issues

states Joseph Glenmullen, M.D., in *Prozac Backlash*.[87] This statement is made more significant when you consider the amount of research hours, energy, and money that has gone into looking for the genes behind schizophrenia and other mental disorders.

While no "schizophrenic gene" has been identified, it is known that schizophrenia runs in families, in that the risk of a relative of a person with schizophrenia becoming schizophrenic is much higher than the one percent risk found in the general population. Children of two parents with schizophrenia have almost a 40 percent chance of becoming schizophrenic; the risk is nearly 50 percent among those who have an identical twin with schizophrenia.[88]

These statistics do not prove a genetic component, however. The incidence of schizophrenia in families does not follow the classic patterns of genetic inheritance. For example, outside the immediate family, incidence is lower than would be expected if a genetic component were involved. In addition, 89 percent of people with schizophrenia do not have a schizophrenic parent, 81 percent do not have a parent or sibling with schizophrenia, and 63 percent have no family history of schizophrenia.[89] Therefore, the most that can accurately be said at this point is that there is a familial vulnerability in schizophrenia. Whether this is environmental, genetic, or some combination of the two has not been determined.

The lack of conformity to the usual genetic pattern suggests that environmental factors play a role. Whatever the source of the familial vulnerability, it sets the stage for environmental factors to trigger the disorder. *Environmental* in this usage simply means not genetic, so toxins, obstetric complications, and nutritional deficiencies from a poor diet, for example, all fall in the environmental category. From the holistic viewpoint, any illness, including schizophrenia, is a combination of vulnerability (whatever the source) and environmental factors that tip the balance of what the system can bear.

Some kind of vulnerability is clearly operational in schizophrenia, given the statistics on the risk with schizophrenia in parents or a twin. The way this vulnerability is viewed depends on one's medical orientation. While genetic researchers focus on the search for a gene abnormality passed down through families, those who understand the electromagnetic field of the human body and how energy functions in health and disease might consider the contribution of an inherited energy imbalance or an energy legacy passed down from generation to generation (see chapter 5).

In any case, genetics or familial vulnerability does not mean "hopeless or incurable," as biochemical researcher William J. Walsh, Ph.D., explains in chapter 4. By considering the 20 other factors cited here and addressing those that you think or discover have relevance to your condition, you decrease your vulnerability and open the way for restoration of your health.

2. Stress

The subject of stress is a natural follow-up to familial vulnerability because it sums up the environmental influences that, in combination with the vulnerability, likely trigger schizophrenia. The rest of the factors cited in this chapter could be called stressors, in that they put stress on the system, add to a person's total stress load, and in so doing increase that person's vulnerability to becoming ill.

When it comes to stress as in a stressful life event, there appears to be no link between such events and the onset of a psychotic episode. In other words, trauma is not enough as a single factor to cause schizophrenia. When combined with other factors, however, it may play a part in tipping the balance into illness.

The effects of chronic stress are also important to consider. Chronic stress wreaks havoc on the body, mind, and spirit and creates a vicious circle. On the physical level, stress drains nutrients and lowers immunity. The nutritional deficiencies result in compromised neurochemistry in the brain, which in turn reduces the body's ability to cope with stress. Lowered immunity also reduces the stress-coping capacity and opens the body to the development of disease. In addition, it creates disturbances in the energy system of the body, which affects all levels of functioning.

People who develop schizophrenia may be compromised when it comes to coping with stressors of all kinds, meaning all environmental influences that place stress on the system, from obstetric complications to viruses or toxins.[90] What a nonschizophrenic might experience as a normal level of stress might be high stress for a person with a predisposition for schizophrenia.

This is a strong argument for reducing the amount of stress in your life, whether through avoidance of known stressful situations, making changes in your circumstances or lifestyle, and/or practicing relaxation techniques. Attending to the rest of the factors in this chapter can significantly reduce your stress load as well.

3. Chemical Toxicity

Although schizophrenia earned the appellation "cancer of the mind" because of the challenge it poses to the medical world, the devastating impact it has on the lives of those affected, and the fear raised in a patient by the "S" word, akin to the fear raised by the "C" word, the phrase may reflect an unwitting truth. Cancer is a disease of toxicity. How much of a role does toxicity play in schizophrenia?

When you consider the model of environmental stressors mounting to the breaking point in someone who is already vulnerable, exposure to toxins is an important factor to address. Proponents of the historical viewpoint that schizophrenia came into existence in the early 1800s or at least that there was a huge increase in the disorder at that time have suggested that the advent or rise may have been due in part to the dramatic increase in environmental toxins resulting from the Industrial Revolution.

Toxic overload places tremendous stress on the body and contributes to the development of disease. Humans today are exposed to an unprecedented number of chemicals. Testing of anyone on Earth, no matter how remote the area in which they live, will reveal that they are carrying at least 250 chemical contaminants in their body fat.[91] The onslaught of chemicals begins in the womb, with the transmission of toxins from the toxic mother to the fetus, and continues with breast-feeding. An infant in the United States or Europe imbibes "the maximum recommended lifetime dose of dioxin" in only six months of nursing. Dioxin, a pesticide by-product, is one of the most toxic substances on Earth.[92] The point is that we start life with an already accumulating toxic load.

In their report, *In Harm's Way—Toxic Threats to Child Development*, the Greater Boston Physicians for Social Responsibility summarize research on lead, mercury, cadmium, manganese, nicotine, pesticides (many of which are commonly used in homes and schools), dioxin and PCBs (polychlorinated biphenyls; both PCBs and dioxin stay in the food chain once they enter it, as they pervasively have), and solvents used in paint, glue, and cleaning products.

The report notes that in one year alone (1997), industrial plants released more than a billion pounds of these chemicals directly into the environment (air, water, and land). Further, almost 75 percent of the top 20 chemicals (those released in the largest quantities) are known or suspected to be neurotoxicants.[93] Neurotoxicants are substances that are toxic to the brain and the nervous system in general, of obvious implication for schizophrenia. Other sources report that of 70,000 different chemicals being used commercially only 10 percent have been tested for their effect on the nervous system.[94] In addition to the pesticides used directly on crops, the chemicals in the air, water, and soil are fully integrated into our food supply.

"Everyday chemicals have the potential to interfere with the metabolism of brain neurotransmitters . . . in a myriad of pathways," states Sherry A. Rogers, M.D., an authority on environmental medicine. "They interfere with synthesis and metabolism, they block receptor sites, poison enzymes, and much more."[95]

As just one example of how this works, consider the hydrazines, a family of chemicals used widely, notably in pesticides, jet fuels, and growth retardants. Hydrazine is sprayed on potatoes to prolong their shelf life. In the body, this chemical blocks serotonin production by blocking the action of vitamin B_6, which is needed at every step in the series of enzyme actions required in the manufacture of serotonin. In just one bag of potato chips or one serving of fast-food French fries, there is sufficient hydrazine to knock out all the B_6 in your body.[96] (Note that vitamin B_6 deficiency has been found in some types of schizophrenia; see the section below on nutrition and chapter 4.)

While we can't avoid toxic exposure entirely, given the state of our planet, avoiding the use of toxic cleaning and other home and garden products, eating organically grown food, drinking pure bottled or filtered water, and avoiding other sources of toxic exposure wherever possible can at least reduce our toxic loads.

 For information on clearing toxins from your body, home, and beyond, see Richard Leviton, *The Healthy Living Space* (Hampton Roads, 2001).

4. Heavy Metal Toxicity

As with chemicals, heavy metals contribute to the toxic burden our bodies are being forced to carry. Examples of heavy metals are mercury, copper, lead, and aluminum. Research has linked all of these to the presence of mental symptoms.[97]

Mercury is well recognized as a neurotoxin, and has been for centuries. Early hatmakers contracted what was known as "mad hatter's disease," the result of poisoning from the mercury used in hatmaking—hence the saying, "mad as a hatter."

Physiologically, mercury's effects on the brain arise from its ability to bond firmly with structures in the nervous system, explains Dr. Dietrich Klinghardt, whose work is featured in chapter 5. Research shows that it is taken up in the peripheral nervous system by all nerve endings (in the tongue, lungs, intestines, and connective tissue, for example) and then transported quickly via nerves to the spinal cord and brainstem.

"Once mercury has traveled up the axon, the nerve cell is impaired in its ability to detoxify itself and in its ability to nurture itself," says Dr. Klinghardt. "The cell becomes toxic and dies—or lives in a state of chronic malnutrition. . . . A multitude of illnesses, usually associated with neurological symptoms, result."[98]

Mercury is bioaccumulative, which means that it doesn't break down in the environment or in the body. The result is that it is everywhere in our environment, in our food, air, and water, and each exposure adds to our internal accumulation. Many of us also carry a source of mercury in our mouths in the form of dental fillings; so-called silver fillings are actually comprised of over 50 percent mercury. These fillings leach mercury, predominantly in the form of vapor, 80 percent of which is absorbed through the lungs into the bloodstream. Chewing raises the level of vapor emission and it remains elevated for at least 90 minutes afterward.[99]

Mercury toxicity can produce a range of symptoms, many of which are associated with schizophrenia. Symptoms include hallucinations, intense anxiety, severe irritability, fits of anger, depression, mania, fatigue, insomnia, sensitivity to stress, headaches, cognitive impairment, lack of concentration, and motor disturbances, among numerous others.[100]

 For information on mercury detoxification, see chapter 5.

Like mercury, copper is found in dental fillings, often added as an alloy to gold fillings. Other sources of copper exposure are cigarettes, cookware, and water pipes. High copper levels in the body have been linked to schizophrenia (see chapter 4).

Lead exposure is often an occupational hazard; approximately one million Americans are exposed to lead on the job.[101] Other sources of exposure include certain glazed ceramics, old paint, water pipes, fertilizers, and soft vinyl products. As with mercury, among the many symptoms of lead toxicity are hallucinations, depression, mania, irritability, insomnia, sensitivity to stress, headaches, cognitive impairment, and motor disturbances, as well as heightened aggression.[102]

Aluminum toxicity has been linked to hallucinations, mental deterioration, motor disturbances, seizures, depression, and Alzheimer's disease, among other conditions and symptoms.[103] Common sources of aluminum exposure are cookware, aluminum salts in baking powder, aluminum-containing antacids, and many antiperspirants and deodorants.

Avoiding exposure to these heavy metals wherever possible both reduces your overall toxic load and removes a potential source of exacerbation of your symptoms. Note that removal of mercury fillings is a stressful procedure for the body and may not be advisable in all cases (see chapter 5).

5. Food Allergies

A discussion of allergies involves what happens in the body on the physical level as well as on the energetic level. On a physical level, eating foods that prompt an immune system reaction (foods to which one is sensitive or allergic) can actually interfere with neurotransmitter function.[104] In terms of energy, allergic reaction is a primary cause of impeded flow of energy through the body, notes allergy authority Devi S. Nambudripad, M.D., D.C., L.Ac., Ph.D. Symptoms of mental illness can result. "Our psychiatric hospitals might be empty if the causes of our energy blockages could be found and removed," she states.[105]

Many people are not aware that they are suffering from food allergies, as the symptoms are often not clearly linked with ingestion of the food, as is the case when someone breaks out in a rash after eating strawberries or experiences a dangerous constriction of air passages after eating shellfish. The allergy goes undetected and the chronic reaction, with its attendant energy blockage, can create a panoply of symptoms, including those of schizophrenia, bipolar disorder, and clinical depression.

Allergies may actually be intolerances or sensitivities resulting from compromised immune and digestive systems or energy disturbances. Once these factors are eliminated or eased, the food intolerances may disappear.

Food intolerances occur when the body doesn't digest food adequately, which results in large undigested protein molecules entering the intestines from the stomach. When poor digestion is chronic, these large molecules push through the lining of the intestines, creating the condition known as leaky gut, and enter the bloodstream. There, these substances are out of context, not recognized as food molecules, and so are regarded as foreign invaders.

The immune system sends an antibody (also called an immunoglobulin) to bind with the foreign protein (antigen), a process which produces the chemicals of allergic response. The antigen-antibody combination is known as a circulating immune complex, or CIC. Normally, a CIC is destroyed or removed from the body, but under conditions of weakened immunity, CICs tend to accumulate in the blood, putting the body on allergic alert, if you will. Thereafter, whenever the person eats the food in question, an allergic reaction follows.

Allergic reactions tend to affect certain organs or meridians in individuals, depending on where their weak or vulnerable areas are, says Dr. Nambudripad. The organ most affected is known as the "target organ." The weakness can be genetic in nature or created by environmental factors such as toxic exposure or lack of adequate nutrition. The target organ can be the nervous system or the brain. If that is the case, chronic allergic reaction can negatively affect brain and nervous system function.

In the case of food allergies, "with the first bite of an allergic food, the brain begins to block the energy channels, attempting to prevent the adverse energy of the food from entering into the body," says Dr. Nambudripad.[106] Chronic blockage of the Stomach meridian (in acupuncture, one of the body's primary energy channels) can also affect brain function. Schizophrenia, manic disorders, and depressive disorders are among the manifestations of this blockage. When the liver is the target organ or the Liver meridian (another of the primary energy channels in acupuncture) is blocked, emotional imbalances, anger, mood swings, and depression are among the outcomes.[107]

As for how the allergies or sensitivities develop in the first place, Dr. Nambudripad cites heredity, toxins, weakened immunity, emotional stress, overexposure to a substance, and radiation. Anything that causes energy blockages in the body, which throws off the body's electromagnetic field, can cause an allergy to develop, she says. Toxins of any kind, from the neurotoxin mercury to the byproducts of bacterial infection, disturb energy flow, as do synthetic food additives and artificial sweeteners.

Until recently, allergies were thought to affect only the mucous membranes, the respiratory tract, and the skin. A growing body of evidence indicates that an allergy can have profound effects on the brain and, as a result, behavior. An allergy or intolerance that affects the brain is known as a brain allergy or a cerebral allergy. Pioneering researcher Carl Pfeiffer, M.D., Ph.D. (see chapter 4), discovered that cerebral allergies were the main cause of symptoms in ten percent of schizophrenics.[108]

> **A growing body of evidence indicates that an allergy can have profound effects on the brain and, as a result, behavior. An allergy or intolerance that affects the brain is known as a brain allergy or a cerebral allergy. Pioneering researcher Carl Pfeiffer, M.D., Ph.D., discovered that cerebral allergies were the main cause of symptoms in ten percent of schizophrenics.**

Gluten (a protein found in wheat and other grains) intolerance is a primary brain allergy and implicated in schizophrenia and bipolar disorder. As Dr. Walsh states in chapter 4, gluten intolerance alone can produce the symptoms of schizophrenia.

Gluten is a protein found in wheat, barley, rye, oats, and other cereal grains, and added to many commercial foods. During digestion, this large protein (consisting of long chains of amino acids) is first broken down into smaller peptides before being further reduced into its amino acid components. Peptides are similar to endorphins, substances that athletes know as the source of "runner's high." The peptide form of gluten is called glutemorphin. It is an opioid, meaning that it has an opium-like effect on brain cells.[109]

Gluten is difficult to digest, and many people develop an intolerance to it. In addition, researchers theorize that incomplete

Grains That Contain Gluten

wheat	semolina
spelt	rye
kamut	oats
teff	barley
triticale	

Foods/Substances That Often Contain Gluten

vinegar	food starch
delicatessen meats	monosodium glutamate
bouillon	(MSG)
dextrin	malt
caramel color	rice syrup
hydrolyzed plant or	natural and artificial flavorings
vegetable protein	

There are many other foods and substances that may contain gluten, including chewing gum, condiments, confectioner's sugar, envelope glue, frozen French fries, ice cream, medications, salad dressings, tomato paste, tuna fish, and vitamin/mineral supplements. Watch for hidden sources of gluten in the diet. Call the manufacturer of a product if you have any doubt.[113]

digestion of gluten leads to excessive absorption of glutemorphins from the intestines into the bloodstream, which leads in turn to their passage across the blood-brain barrier where they exert their opioid effects.[110] In so doing, they depress serotonin, dopamine, and norepinephrine levels in the brain.[111] Research has found that when people who are sensitive to gluten eat food containing it, their neurological function is altered.[112]

Avoidance of allergens is one way to prevent allergic reactions, but many people are allergic to ubiquitous substances or do not even know to what they are allergic. NAET (Nambudripad's Allergy Elimination Techniques) is a painless, effective method for both identifying and eliminating allergies.

For more about NAET, see chapter 5. For more about allergies, see chapters 3 and 5.

Allergy elimination can be beneficial for schizophrenia in several ways: (1) directly, by removing the source of allergy-related symptoms of schizophrenia; and (2) indirectly, by easing other problems that may be exacerbating or producing symptoms. In the latter category, eliminating allergic reaction improves digestion, which can help reverse the nutrient assimilation and absorption problems that may be contributing to the deficiencies associated with schizophrenia.

Increased absorption of all nutrients will improve the health of all body systems. Getting rid of allergic reaction also reduces toxic substances in the body, which lifts a burden from the liver and other parts of the detoxification system, leading to more optimal processing of toxins in the future. Finally, allergy elimination lifts a large burden from the immune system, which increases resistance and leads to better overall health.

6. Intestinal Dysbiosis

Intestinal dysbiosis means an imbalance of the flora that normally inhabit the intestines. Among the many types of these flora are the beneficial bacteria (known as probiotics) *Lactobacillus acidophilus* and *Bifidobacterium bifidum,* potentially harmful bacteria such as *E. coli* and *Clostridium,* and the fungus *Candida albicans.* When the balance among intestinal flora is disturbed, the microorganisms held in check by the beneficial bacteria proliferate and release toxins that compromise intestinal function. This has far-reaching effects in the body and on the mind.

Research has revealed that what passes through the lining of the intestines (see Food Allergies) can make its way through the bloodstream to the brain.[114] As an example of just one of the results of this relationship, in the brain, certain intestinal bacteria can interfere with neurotransmitter function.[115]

Dysbiosis contributes to a buildup of toxins in the body in two ways. One, the harmful bacteria's normal metabolism processes release toxic by-products. Two, a compromised intestinal system cannot adequately filter toxins, which is one of the important functions of the intestinal lining. Normally, bile from the liver goes through the intestines where toxins are filtered out, and the bile is then recirculated, cleansed. When the intestines are not working correctly, bile is returned to the body with the old toxicity. This condition is known as enterohepatic toxicity (*entero* for intestines and *hepatic* for liver). Toxic buildup compromises the functioning of the entire system, including the brain.

Depression, fatigue, anxiety, irritability, agitation, memory and concentration problems, dizziness, insomnia, headaches, feelings of unreality, and even delusions, mania, psychosis, and suicidal or violent tendencies are among the symptoms that can result from candidiasis, an overgrowth of *Candida albicans,* the yeast-like fungus normally found in the body.[116] Mercury is often implicated in this overgrowth because "the purpose of *Candida* in the human being is to protect the body from mercury by absorbing it," says Thomas M. Rau, M.D., director of the Paracelsus Klinik in Lustmühle, Switzerland. The mechanism was never intended, however, to deal with large amounts of mercury. Nevertheless, when mercury levels in the body are high, the population of *Candida* multiplies in a vain attempt to deal with the heavy metal load.

Through its normal metabolic processes, *Candida* releases substances that are toxic to the brain and interfere with neurotransmitter activity.[117] Another mechanism by which *Candida* overgrowth has an impact on the brain is that the intestinal lining becomes inflamed, which interferes with the absorption of nutrients.[118] As discussed later, nutritional deficiencies are implicated in schizophrenia.

Candida overgrowth occurs when something intervenes to disturb the normal balance of flora in the intestinal environment. The main culprit in throwing off the balance is antibiotics, particularly the repeated use of antibiotics, which kill all the beneficial bacteria that keep potentially harmful flora such as *Candida* in check. Weakened immunity may also be a factor in yeast overgrowth.

Eliminating foods that "feed" *Candida* is a common treatment approach to restoring intestinal balance. The so-called *Candida* diet emphasizes avoiding all forms and sources of sugar, including fruit and fruit juice, carbohydrates, and fermented yeast products. According to Dr. Rau, however, the relationship between mercury and *Candida* means that until you detoxify the body of the mercury, you won't be able to get rid of the *Candida* overgrowth on any lasting basis, no matter how perfect your diet or what antifungal drug or natural substance you take. The fungus will just keep coming back.[119]

In addition to antibiotics, anti-inflammatory drugs, food allergies, and a poor diet can all help create intestinal dysbiosis.

7. Sensitivity to Food Additives

Research has established that aspartame (an artificial sweetener), aspartic acid (an amino acid in aspartame), glutamic acid (found in flavor enhancers and salt substitutes), and the artificial flavoring MSG (monosodium glutamate) are neurotoxins.[120] Aspartame alters amino acid ratios and blocks serotonin production.[121] MSG has been shown to affect serotonin levels.[122]

The more than 3,000 additives used in commercially prepared food have not been tested by their manufacturers for their effects on the nervous system or on behavior.[123] In addition to those mentioned, common food additives are artificial flavoring, artificial preservatives (BHA, BHT, and TBHQ are in this category), artificial coloring/food dyes, thickeners, moisteners, and artificial sweeteners.

According to reports to the FDA (Food and Drug Administration), complaints associated with ingestion of aspartame include hypersensitivity to noise, ringing or buzzing in the ears, vision problems, gastrointestinal problems, irritability, and depression.[124] Other symptoms linked to food additives are restlessness, sleep disturbance, and distractibility.[125]

Sensitivity to food additives varies; a high sensitivity may reflect an already large toxic load or weakened immunity. Noticing if your symptoms worsen after ingesting certain foods can start the process of elimination for determining which additives, if any, are problematic for you.

8. Nutritional Deficiencies and Imbalances

Nutritional deficiencies and imbalances are a common feature in schizophrenia and other mental illnesses. Correcting these often produces dramatic improvement. Unfortunately, nutrient status testing and intervention are not standard practice in conventional psychiatric medicine. "Nutrient related disorders are always treatable and deficiencies are usually curable. To ignore their existence is tantamount to malpractice," states Richard A. Kunin, M.D.,[126] a practitioner of orthomolecular medicine (see chapter 3).

No two people with schizophrenia will have the exact same nutritional condition. Blood chemistry analysis can determine the precise status of your nutrient levels. With this information, therapeutic intervention can then be tailored to your specific nutrient needs. Random supplementation may not address those needs and may even contribute to further skewing of nutrient ratios.

While other factors such as absorption problems or even a genetic disorder may be involved in nutritional deficiencies and imbalances, poor diet is a primary cause. Any factor that contributes to your vulnerability should be avoided if you suffer from schizophrenia. Erratic eating habits or a nutrient-depleted diet, as in junk-food, fast-food, processed-food diets, definitely fall into the category of contributing to vulnerability. Feeding the brain and nervous system the nutrients they require to function properly is a basic building block of health.

There are several general principles to consider in the issue of nutrition and schizophrenia. The first is true for everyone, and that is that the more toxins there are in your environment, the greater will be your nutritional needs in order for your body to defend against them. The second is that the nutritional needs of schizophrenia are already higher than they are for other people.

The nutritional issues of schizophrenia are discussed at length in chapters 3 and 4, but here we look briefly at the main areas of concern, which are essential fatty acids, vitamins B and C, and certain minerals.

Essential Fatty Acids

Research has discovered a link between lipids and mental disorders. Lipids are fats or oils, which are comprised of fatty acids. Examples of saturated fatty acids are animal fats and other fats, such as coconut oil, that are solid at room temperature. Examples of unsaturated fatty acids, which remain liquid at room temperature, are certain plant and fish oils. Essential fatty acids (EFAs) are unsaturated fats required for many metabolic actions in the body.

There are two main types of EFAs: omega 3 and omega 6. The primary omega-3 EFAs are: ALA (alpha-linolenic acid); DHA (docosahexaenoic acid); and EPA (eicosapentaenoic acid). ALA is found in flaxseed and canola oils, pumpkins, walnuts, and soybeans, while DHA and EPA are found in the oils of cold-water fish such as salmon, cod, and mackerel.

Two important types of omega-6 EFAs are GLA (gamma-linolenic acid) and linoleic acid or cis-linoleic acid. Evening primrose, black currant, and borage oils are sources of GLA, while linoleic acid is found in most plants and vegetable oils, notably safflower, corn, peanut, and sesame oils. The body converts omega-3 and omega-6 EFAs into prostaglandins, which are hormone-like substances involved in many metabolic functions.

The ratio of omega-3 to omega-6 EFAs is skewed in the standard American diet, which is deficient in omega 3s. High consumption of hydrogenated oils and beef contributes to the skewed ratio. Hydrogenated oils (which are oils processed to extend shelf life) are detrimental in two ways: not only does refining oil reduce its omega-3 content, but hydrogenated oils also take up the fatty acid receptor sites and interfere with normal fatty acid metabolism. Hydrogenated oils, also known as trans-fatty acids, are found in margarine, commercial baked goods, crackers, cookies, and other products. The problem with conventionally raised beef cattle is that they are grain-fed rather than grass-fed; grain is high in omega 6 and low in omega 3, while grass provides a more balanced ratio.[127]

Andrew Stoll, M.D., a psychopharmacology researcher and an assistant professor of psychiatry at Harvard Medical School, states: "Omega-3 fatty acids . . . are essential nutrients for human brain development and general health. Over the past 50 to 100 years, there has been an accelerated deficiency of omega-3 fatty acids in most Western countries. There is emerging evidence that this progressive omega-3 deficiency is responsible, at least in part, for the rise in the incidence of heart disease, asthma, bipolar disorder, major depression, and perhaps autism."[128] (Note that in certain cases of schizophrenia, those involving a condition called pyroluria, the EFA that is deficient is omega-6; see chapter 4.)

Lipids are necessary for the health of the blood vessels that feed the brain and comprise 50 to 60 percent of the brain's solid matter.[129] More specifically, nerve cells in the brain contain high levels of omega-3 fatty acids.[130] A deficiency could obviously have serious consequences.

A review of the research on omega-3 EFAs concluded that there is substantial evidence to indicate that they may play a role in schizophrenia.[131] One study found that schizophrenics had low levels of arachidonic acid, linoleic acid, EPA, and DHA compared to nonschizophrenics. Just six weeks of EFA supplementation resulted in a marked raising of those levels as well as a "significant decrease" in symptom severity. In addition, those with a higher intake of EFAs before the study had less severe symptoms to start with than did those with a lower intake. The researchers noted that the diets of the subjects were not deficient in EFAs. From this, they concluded that EFA metabolism dysfunction rather than pure deficiency is the problem connected to schizophrenia.[132]

Vitamins and Minerals

As you can see from the list of psychological and emotional symptoms of deficiency in the accompanying sidebar, the vitamin B family is essential for mental health. The link between B vitamins and the mind is clear in the disease called pellagra, which mimics schizophrenia and is caused by a deficiency of vitamin B_3 (niacin). This disease was common in the 1930s before the advent of vitamin-enriched bread.[133]

Based on the clinical experience of the practitioners in this book, the most common vitamin deficiencies associated with schizophrenia are vitamin B_3 (niacin/niacinamide), vitamin B_6 (pyridoxine), B_{12} (cobalamin), and folic acid (a member of the

Psychological/Emotional Effects of Vitamin Deficiencies

The following are psychological/emotional symptoms that can result from deficiencies in vitamin C and the B-complex vitamin family.

Deficient Vitamin	Resulting Behavior
Ascorbic acid (vitamin C)	Hysteria, confusion, depression, lassitude, hypochondriasis
Biotin	Depression, extreme lassitude, somnolence
Folic acid	Insomnia, irritability, forgetfulness, depression, apathy, delirium, dementia, psychosis
Vitamin B_1 (thiamin)	Apathy, anxiety, irritability, depression, memory loss, personality changes, emotional instability
Vitamin B_2 (riboflavin)	Depression, insomnia, mental sluggishness
Vitamin B_3 (niacin/niacinamide)	Apathy, anxiety, depression, mania, hyperirritability, emotional instability, memory and concentration problems
Vitamin B_5 (pantothenic acid)	Restlessness, irritability, fatigue, depression, quarrelsomeness
Vitamin B_6 (pyridoxine)	Irritability, nervousness, insomnia, poor dream recall, depression
Vitamin B_{12} (cobalamin)	Mood swings, depression, irritability, confusion, memory loss, hallucinations, delusions, paranoia, psychotic states

Source: Adapted by permission of Rita Elkins, from her book Depression and Natural Medicine: A Nutritional Approach to Depression and Mood Swings *(Pleasant Grove, Utah: Woodland Publishing, 1995): 75.*

vitamin B family), all of which are vital to neurotransmitter function. Biochemical researcher William Walsh, Ph.D., has found that a genetic disorder, which causes severe deficiency in both vitamin B_6 and zinc, can be a factor in schizophrenia (see chapter 4).

Vitamin C is also vital to neurotransmitter function. A number of research findings are of interest in regard to vitamin C and schizophrenia, notably: (1) the blood levels of vitamin C are often low in schizophrenics; (2) the point at which their bodies reach saturation when taking vitamin C is 12 to 16 times higher than it is for nonschizophrenics, which resembles the situation with people who suffer from scurvy (a disease caused by vitamin C deficiency); and (3) in populations with a low intake of vitamin C the incidence of schizophrenia is higher than in populations with a higher intake.[134]

Of minerals, zinc is the mineral most often found deficient, while manganese and magnesium are of importance as supplements in treating certain categories of schizophrenia, as is discussed in chapter 4. For example, magnesium enhances vitamin B_6 activity and, taken as a supplement, helps prevent the magnesium deficiency that can result from high doses of B_6.

Poor diet and malabsorption due to gastrointestinal dysfunction are common causes of nutritional deficiencies. The depleted mineral content of the soil in which crops are grown, which translates into food with a lower mineral content than our forebears enjoyed, is a factor as well. Finally, many lifestyle practices and attributes of modern life deplete us of vitamins and minerals, regardless of how well we eat: stress, smoking, alcohol, caffeine, pollution, and heavy metals such as the mercury in our dental fillings.

Given these factors, the recommended daily allowance (RDA; purportedly, the amount of individual vitamins and minerals our body requires daily, whether from food or supplements) is likely far below our nutritive needs, in most cases. The RDA standard is based on a group norm for preventing nutritional deficiencies. There are two problems with that. One, individual needs diverge widely, and two, the level of deficiency the RDAs are designed to avoid is severe. The systems of the body can begin to be compromised long before that degree of deficiency registers. In other words, if you use the RDAs as your guideline, you could be walking around with moderate nutritional deficiencies, especially given the higher nutritional needs or malfunction of nutrient systems found in schizophrenia.

While increasing your intake of foods that contain the nutrients cited is unlikely to reverse deficiencies, it can serve as an adjunct to supplementation. The following are dietary sources of these nutrients:

- Vitamin B$_3$: brewer's yeast, rice bran, peanuts, eggs, milk, fish, legumes, avocado, liver and other organ meats

- Vitamin B$_6$: brewer's yeast, wheat germ, bananas, seeds, nuts, legumes, avocado, leafy green vegetables, potatoes, cauliflower, chicken, whole grains

- Vitamin B$_{12}$: liver, kidneys, eggs, clams, oysters, fish, dairy

- Folic acid: brewer's yeast, green leafy vegetables, wheat germ, soybeans, legumes, asparagus, broccoli, oranges, sunflower seeds

- Vitamin C: green vegetables (particularly broccoli, Brussels sprouts, green peppers, kale, turnip greens, and collards), fruits (particularly guava, persimmons, black currants, strawberries, papaya, and citrus; citrus contains less vitamin C than the other fruits)

- Zinc: oysters, herring, sunflower seeds, pumpkin seeds, lima beans, legumes, soybeans, wheat germ, brewer's yeast, dairy

- Magnesium: parsnips, tofu, buckwheat, beans, leafy green vegetables, wheat germ, blackstrap molasses, kelp, brewer's yeast, nuts, seeds, bananas, avocado, dairy, seafood

- Manganese: whole grains (especially buckwheat and bulgur), nuts, sunflower seeds, leafy green vegetables

9. Neurotransmitter Deficiencies or Dysfunction

The neurotransmitters seemingly most implicated in schizophrenia—dopamine, serotonin, epinephrine/norepinephrine,

GABA, and glutamate—are discussed in chapter 1. The theory that a problem with these brain chemicals is behind schizophrenia has not been proven, and even the nature of the problem is unclear.

It used to be thought that it was merely a matter of supply, but research now indicates that the issue is more complicated. A normal level of a given neurotransmitter does not guarantee that the mind and body will receive its benefits. For example, despite high blood levels of the neurotransmitter serotonin, reduced uptake in the brain may mean that the availability of this vital nerve messenger is actually limited.[135] One school of thought holds that the problem in schizophrenia is more likely dysfunction in the complex connections linking different regions of the brain, connections that occur via neurotransmitters.[136]

Amino acids are the basic building blocks for neurotransmitters. The body does not manufacture most of the amino acids it requires, so they must be obtained through protein in the diet. With a deficient diet, the body is not able to produce sufficient neurotransmitters. While supplementation with the amino acid precursors to neurotransmitters has been found to be highly beneficial in bipolar disorder, the same cannot be said of schizophrenia. This may be a reflection of the need for more investigation.

In any case, attempting to correct neurotransmitter supply or even function does not address the root problem of why the supply is low or the neurotransmitters are not working properly. As you will learn in part 2 of this book, treating the root imbalances involved in a particular individual's schizophrenia can result in a resolution of symptoms. When enough of the factors interfering with the body's natural balance are removed, the body is restored to its innate ability to heal itself.

10. Structural Factors

Structural factors such as cranial compression can be a component in schizophrenia. Such compression, which is the result of skull distortion, can occur through birth trauma or a later physical trauma, such as a car accident. Research has linked obstetric complications to an increased risk of schizophrenia,[137] and seven studies have found that subjects with schizophrenia had a statistically higher incidence of obstetrical complications during their birth.[138]

The impact of cranial compression has far-reaching effects throughout the body, but in the head the compression exerts pressure on the brain and cranial nerves, which compromises neurotransmitter function and brain function in general. This factor and its treatment are explored in depth in chapter 6.

11. Viruses

Researchers have long been exploring a possible connection between viruses and schizophrenia. While a viral cause has not been identified, viruses are implicated in a number of ways: (1) a prenatal exposure to flu is associated with an increased risk of schizophrenia;[139] (2) people with schizophrenia are more likely to have been born in the winter or early spring, that is, the flu season;[140] and (3) increases in the rate of schizophrenia have been shown to occur 20 to 30 years after severe flu epidemics, with the rate returning to normal thereafter.[141]

With the knowledge of a prenatal viral exposure, it becomes even more important to reduce other environmental stressors that may in combination trigger the development of schizophrenia.

In addition to viral factors that may contribute to schizophrenia, certain viral infections can mimic the symptoms of schizophrenia. These include viral encephalitis, herpes simplex, Epstein-Barr, cytomegalovirus, measles, coxsackie, and human immunodeficiency virus (HIV).[142]

 For more about viruses and schizophrenia, see chapter 5.

12. Hypoglycemia

Hypoglycemia, commonly known as low blood sugar, is a condition in which the glucose level in the blood is lower than normal. The brain relies upon a stable glucose supply for its functioning and the symptoms of low blood sugar are an immediate reflection of a deficit. They include restlessness, irritability, fatigue, impairment of mental functions, and, when severe, mental disturbances including those that occur in schizophrenia.[143]

The fact that hypoglycemia is not generally considered in the treatment of schizophrenia is an unfortunate oversight because most people with schizophrenia suffer from hypoglycemia, and the rate of diabetes (which also involves glucose metabolism problems) is high as well.[144]

As unstable blood sugar may contribute to or exacerbate your symptoms, you may want to consult with your doctor and eliminate hypoglycemia as a factor in your schizophrenia.

13. Hormonal Imbalances

Hormones "are probably second only to the chemicals of the brain in shaping how we feel and behave."[145] Hormonal imbalances influence brain chemistry and the nervous system,[146] as neurons are extremely sensitive to shifts in their hormonal environment.[147]

Hormonal imbalances involving thyroid or adrenal hormones can produce symptoms similar enough to schizophrenia that misdiagnosis can occur. The primary adrenal hormones are cortisol, DHEA, epinephrine, and norepinephrine. Given the role of the latter two as neurotransmitters and ones thought to play a part in schizophrenia, the implications of imbalance are clear.

Cushing's syndrome is a specific adrenal gland malfunction

> **The fact that hypoglycemia is not generally considered in the treatment of schizophrenia is an unfortunate oversight because most people with schizophrenia suffer from hypoglycemia, and the rate of diabetes (which also involves glucose metabolism problems) is high as well. As unstable blood sugar may contribute to or exacerbate your symptoms, you may want to consult with your doctor and eliminate hypoglycemia as a factor in your schizophrenia.**

that results in excessive production of glucocorticoids, adrenal hormones that protect against stress and play a role in protein and carbohydrate metabolism. This disorder can produce delusions and hallucinations and is one of the medical conditions sometimes mistaken for schizophrenia.[148]

Hypo- and hyperthyroidism (an underactive and overactive thyroid, respectively) are two thyroid conditions that can produce psychotic symptoms (delusions or hallucinations) that can be mistaken for schizophrenia. Hypothyroidism is often overlooked as a cause because it can be at a subclinical level and still produce symptoms.

On the positive side of hormonal influences on schizophrenia, it may be that estrogen, one of the reproductive hormones, exerts an antipsychotic effect. The theory of the protective quality of estrogen is supported by the fact that schizophrenia is more common and tends to be more severe among men, and that women with schizophrenia tend to relapse when estrogen is low, as during menopause and after giving birth. In addition, one study found that estrogen replacement therapy reduced psychotic symptoms.[149]

There are many causes of hormonal imbalance. Toxic exposure, stress, diet, and exercise can all affect hormonal levels and balance. If you suspect that you have a hormonal imbalance of some kind, consult with your doctor about it. If you discover that there is indeed a problem, it is advisable to work with a natural medicine practitioner to correct the imbalances, rather than take synthetic hormones. The latter can be detrimental to your health, so it is best to avoid them if possible.

14. Medical Conditions

According to the *DSM-IV*, the following medical conditions can produce psychotic symptoms that can be mistaken for schizophrenia: brain tumor, Huntington's disease, cerebrovascular disease, multiple sclerosis, epilepsy, central nervous system infections, migraine, impairment of auditory or visual nerves, Cushing's syndrome (see Hormonal Imbalances), hyper- and hypothyroidism (see Hormonal Imbalances), hypoglycemia (see earlier section), hypercarbia (higher than normal levels of carbon dioxide in the blood), hypoxia (oxygen deficiency), electrolyte or fluid imbalances, liver or kidney disease, and lupus and other autoimmune disorders that involve the central nervous system.[150]

Certain viral infections can also mimic symptoms (see earlier section), as can syphilis. Pellagra, which is caused by a niacin deficiency and used to be quite common, is another disorder that resembles schizophrenia (see Nutritional Deficiencies and Imbalances).

15. Medications

A relatively new diagnostic category in the *DSM-IV* is Substance-Induced Psychotic Disorder. In this case, hallucinations and delusions are caused by medications or street drugs. Among the medications cited is methylphenidate (Ritalin).[151] This is alarming given the wanton prescription of Ritalin to children in the United States.

The *DSM-IV* also cites the following as sources of drug-induced psychosis: antipsychotics, anxiolytics, anticholinergics, antiparkinsonian medications, anticonvulsants, barbiturates (sedatives and hypnotics), benzodiazepines (tranquilizers and sleeping pills), analgesics (pain relievers), anesthetics, antihypertensives (for high blood pressure), antiulcer medications, heart medications, oral contraceptives, muscle relaxants, corticosteroids (prednisone and cortisone are in this category), antihistamines, and nonsteroidal anti-inflammatory drugs (NSAIDs; ibuprofen is in this category), among others.[152]

Note that antipsychotics and other drugs used for schizophrenia are included in this list. Yes, the very drugs prescribed for schizophrenia can produce psychotic symptoms. Dr. Abram Hoffer, whose work is covered in chapter 3, calls this "tranquilizer psychosis." This is a secondary psychosis that develops with long-term use of antipsychotic drugs.

It is well known that certain antidepressant drugs can also

induce psychosis. A common belief is that this is only a danger with the older classes of antidepressants, that the newer SSRIs (selective serotonin re-uptake inhibitors) such as Prozac are free of this problem. Unfortunately, this is not the case. One study found, for example, that the psychosis or mania of 43 out of 533 patients admitted to a psychiatric hospital was connected to anti-depressant use, and 70 percent of those patients were on Prozac, Zoloft, Paxil, or another SSRI.[153]

16. Street Drugs

As with prescription medications, street drugs can also induce psychosis that resembles and can be misdiagnosed as schiz-ophrenia. The drugs most commonly implicated are ampheta-mines, cocaine (and crack), phencyclidine (PCP or angel dust), marijuana, and hallucinogens such as LSD.

For people who are indeed schizophrenic, use of street drugs, particularly PCP, marijuana, and stimulants such as ampheta-mines and cocaine, worsens symptoms and the outcome of the ill-ness.[154] In addition, use of stimulants or PCP increases the likelihood of the person becoming violent.[155] Dr. E. Fuller Torrey describes such drugs as "like poison for anyone with schizophre-nia."[156]

17. Caffeine, Alcohol, and Nicotine

In the general population, people who drink a lot of coffee test higher for anxiety and depression and are also more likely than their more abstemious counterparts to develop psychotic dis-orders.[157] Among psychiatric patients, research has found that the level of caffeine ingested is positively correlated with the degree of mental illness,[158] meaning that the more caffeine taken in, the worse the symptoms.

Caffeine does a lot more than give you a jittery edge. It actu-ally affects your neurotransmitters, stimulating the release of nor-epinephrine and others. Habitual excess intake can leave you with a neurotransmitter deficit, along with hypoglycemia and nutritional deficiencies, as it interferes with the absorption of important nutrients such as B vitamins, magnesium, calcium, potassium, and zinc.[159] Note the overlap with nutritional deficiencies often present in schizophrenia.

Avoiding caffeine or at least limiting intake is thus advisable. Be sure to consider all caffeine sources. Some people give up or cut down on coffee and black tea, but overlook the high caffeine content in colas.

Alcohol also interferes with normal neurotransmitter function by impeding the supply of tryptophan to the brain and thus reducing serotonin formation. As with caffeine, habitual drinking of alcoholic beverages is associated with hypoglycemia and nutritional deficiencies, notably B vitamins, vitamin C, folic acid, zinc, potassium, and magnesium.[160] Finally, as with street drugs, drinking increases the likelihood of the person with schizophrenia becoming violent.[161]

As noted in chapter 1, the rate of cigarette smoking is very high among people with schizophrenia; 80 to 90 percent smoke. The reasons for this are as numerous as they are among smokers in the general population, but there is one effect of nicotine that has particular relevance for people with schizophrenia. Research indicates that smoking reduces the function of antipsychotic drugs; smokers need higher doses compared to nonsmokers to produce the same level of effect.[162] Smoking may also reduce the Parkinsonian-like side effects of antipsychotic drugs and provide temporary improvement in the symptoms of mental impairment associated with schizophrenia.[163]

While this may sound like support for smoking, there are many more reasons in support of quitting or at least cutting back. In addition to the known health hazards posed by smoking, nicotine, like stimulants and alcohol, affects neurotransmitters. In the brain, it behaves like acetylcholine, excess levels of which may worsen psychotic symptoms and have been linked to anxiety, irritability, muscle twitching, and seizures.[164]

18. Lack of Sleep

Sleep deprivation is known to produce psychotic symptoms. One of the warning signs of relapse for many people with schizophrenia is a change in sleep patterns. Aside from this, sufficient sleep supports balance at all levels of one's being. It is as important as a healthful diet. Getting enough sleep and avoiding the stress that "all-nighters" place on the body and mind is another way to lighten the environmental load, which when too heavy may tip into psychosis.

19. Lack of Exercise

Exercise stimulates the release of mood-regulating epinephrine, norepinephrine, and serotonin, along with endorphins, chemicals that lift our mood and reduce our stress level. It increases oxygen, glucose, and nutrient supply to the brain, which improves cerebral function and the ability to cope with stress.[165] Exercise also helps flush toxins out of the body, the benefits of which were discussed previously.

Exercise can alleviate schizophrenic symptoms, irritability, insomnia, depression, anxiety, and hyperactivity.[166] As with food and sleep, it is a basic need of the body. Lack of exercise is an environmental stressor that is relatively easy to remedy.

20. Energy Imbalances

There are a number of different ways to discuss the flow of energy in the human body. Physiologically, the salient point for schizophrenia is that the nervous system operates on electrical charges. Extending outward, you could speak of the body's electromagnetic field and the far-reaching effects on mental and physical health caused by disturbances in that field (see chapter 5).

If you regard energy from the perspective of homeopathy, which is an energy-based medicine, illness is regarded as a disturbance in the individual's vital (life) force. Homeopathic remedies restore that vital force to its natural equilibrium, which restores balance to the body, mind, and spirit (see chapter 7). If you consider energy from a shamanic viewpoint, you might explore the presence of foreign energy in an individual's energy field (see chapter 9).

Whatever language you choose to employ to describe the phenomenon, a disturbance in an individual's energy field can contribute to schizophrenia. The relationship of energy to other factors can be cyclical, with physical factors (such as nutritional deficiencies) or psychological or spiritual issues causing or

> ## In Their Own Words
>
> *"In the most recently published book I've read, a doctor writes that psychotherapy is useless with schizophrenics. . . . [My therapist] is not afraid to travel with me in my fearful times. She listens when I need to release some of the 'poisons' in my mind. She offers advice when I'm having difficulty with just daily living. . . . Psychotherapy is important to me, and it does help."[167]*
>
> —An artist, 37, who suffers from paranoid schizophrenia

being caused by a disturbance in energy flow. As mentioned in the earlier section on familial vulnerability, an inherited energy imbalance or an energy legacy passed down from generation to generation may also be operational (see chapter 5).

21. Psychospiritual Issues

In an article published in the *Psychiatric Times Journal* in December 1996, psychiatrist David Kaiser, M.D., criticized the current solely biological approach to mental illness. "What is left completely out," he wrote, "are any notions that our psychic ills are a reflection of cultural pathology. In fact, this new biologic psychiatry can only exist to the extent it can deny not only the truths of psychoanalysis, but also the truth of any serious cultural criticism. It is then no surprise that this psychiatry thrives in this country presently, where such denials are rampant and deeply embedded."[168]

Support for exploring psychospiritual (psychological and

spiritual) factors in schizophrenia does not mean a return to blaming the disorder on parenting, as was the case during the era when the schizophrenogenic-mother theory was dominant. It is an attempt to restore some balance to the pharmacological age in psychiatric treatment where drugs alone are viewed as the answer.

People are not only their neurotransmitters. Humans are as complex and as much a mystery as schizophrenia is. To ignore the psychological, emotional, and spiritual factors in any illness is to treat only part of a person. As noted in the previous section, these factors have the capacity to throw the energy system out of balance, which can have repercussions on all levels, including the electrical transmission of the nervous system. Thus, treatment that does not address all areas will not produce lasting health.

While psychological trauma alone is not the source of schizophrenia, it can contribute to the total environmental load. The role of psychological stress in schizophrenia is highlighted by the fact that relapse often follows arguments and tension in the person's family.[169] This reflects the impaired ability of schizophrenics to handle stimulation and stress.

Psychotherapy is one avenue for exploring the psychological and spiritual dimensions of your schizophrenia. Aside from the causal contributions in these areas, psychotherapy can provide an important forum for processing all the issues that arise from being diagnosed with and living with schizophrenia. It could be considered as psychological and spiritual housecleaning or the maintenance work that taking good care of something requires. Taking good care of yourself means attending to the needs of body, mind, and spirit.

Psychotherapy is neglected as a component in today's drug-focused treatment despite the fact that research has shown that the addition of psychotherapy and family education to drug treatment makes it possible to lower the dosages of antipsychotic medications.[170]

This research may be related to why people in cultures where extended families are the norm recover better from schizophrenia than those in cultures where extended families are not the norm. Love and care may be the issue at the heart of this, and psychiatric drugs cannot take their place.

Psychosomatic medicine, a European medical discipline that recognizes the role and interrelationship of body, mind, and spirit in mental and physical health, is another modality for dealing with psychospiritual disturbances. Chapter 8 explores this discipline's approach to schizophrenia.

Shamanic healing addresses both energy disturbances and the psychic or spiritual issues that may be involved in an individual's schizophrenia. The shamanic view of mental illness provides valuable insight, as it is entirely different from the way in which the Western world regards such disorders. The shamanic view and shamanic healing are thoroughly discussed in chapter 9.

Schizophrenia is a complex condition. No single factor is responsible for creating it in everyone and no single therapeutic measure can reverse it in everyone. To look for the single cause of schizophrenia, as is often the focus in conventional research, is to ignore the many factors that can be addressed now, even without establishing a definitive causal link. If correcting or addressing a factor or factors discussed in this chapter produces improvement or even reversal of schizophrenic symptoms, that is sufficient reason for doing so. Although it doesn't prove that the factors caused the person's schizophrenia, it indicates that they at least contributed.

While most people will not have all 21 of the factors in operation, having more than a few, especially those that directly affect the biochemistry of the brain, may be sufficient to cause psychotic symptoms, depending on the individual's constitution and the severity of the imbalance. In addition to the potential impact on a person's schizophrenia, addressing any of the factors that are operational is an investment in one's health on all levels. Left untreated, these underlying imbalances may produce further physical and mental problems.

All of this underlines the importance of identifying what underlying imbalances are operational in an individual with schizophrenia. By systematically identifying and addressing each one, it is possible to sidestep the issue of causality and simply attend to restoring the individual's health on all levels—body, mind, and spirit. Part 2 of the book explores this approach in depth.

Action Plan

As a summary of the information in this chapter, the following are steps you can take to eliminate or reduce the factors that may be contributing to or exacerbating your schizophrenia.

- Reduce the amount of stress in your life, through avoidance of known stressful situations, making changes in your circumstances or lifestyle, and/or the use of relaxation techniques.

- Reduce your toxic exposure wherever possible. Avoid using toxic house and garden products; eat organically grown food; and drink pure water instead of tap water.

- Reduce your heavy metal exposure by avoiding sources of copper, lead, aluminum, and mercury wherever possible. You may want to investigate having your mercury dental fillings replaced with non-mercury amalgams; hair analysis and other tests can determine if the level of mercury in your body is high.

- Avoid foods and other substances to which you are allergic, or get allergy treatment such as NAET to eliminate the problem (see chapter 5). If you suspect you have allergies, but don't know to what, NAET can help you identify allergens.

- Address any intestinal or digestive dysfunction, such as an overgrowth of *Candida*. Taking probiotics helps improve digestion.

- Avoid food additives, particularly if your symptoms seem to worsen after ingesting additives.

- Eat a healthful, balanced diet. Avoid junk food, fast food, and processed food.

- Have your biochemical status checked to identify any nutritional deficiencies or imbalances, and work with a qualified practitioner to start an appropriate supplement program to correct them (see chapters 3 and 4).

- Have your essential fatty acid levels checked and take the appropriate EFA supplements to correct any imbalances or deficiencies (see chapter 4).

- Consider consulting a cranial osteopath to eliminate structural factors such as cranial compression that may be contributing to your schizophrenia (see chapter 6).

- Consult with your doctor about hypoglycemia. If you have this condition, there are dietary practices you can follow to correct it.

- Have your doctor check for hormonal imbalances if appropriate. If there is a problem, work with a natural medicine practitioner to correct the imbalances. Synthetic hormones can be detrimental to your health, so it is best to avoid them if possible.

- Consult with your doctor to determine if you have any medical conditions that produce schizophrenic symptoms, including viral infections.

- Consult your doctor about whether any medications you are taking might be contributing to your schizophrenia.

- Avoid recreational drugs, particularly cocaine, amphetamines, marijuana, and PCP.

- Limit intake of alcohol, caffeine, and nicotine.

- Get sufficient sleep. Try to avoid "all-nighters."

- Get regular exercise.

- Address energy imbalances through homeopathy or other forms of energy medicine (see chapters 5, 7, and 9).

- Explore psychospiritual issues through psychotherapy or other modalities (see chapters 5, 8, and 9).

Part II

Natural Medicine Treatments for Schizophrenia

3 Orthomolecular Psychiatry

Abram Hoffer, M.D., Ph.D., is one of the founding fathers of orthomolecular medicine. He is responsible for the discovery that niacin lowers cholesterol, which led to a paradigm shift in mainstream medicine. Prior to his research findings, vitamins were considered only for prevention of deficiency diseases such as scurvy (caused by vitamin C deficiency). Subsequent studies clearly demonstrated the role of nutritional supplements in treatment of a range of conditions. In the field of mental disorders, Dr. Hoffer's pioneering work in the treatment of schizophrenia, specifically with megadoses of vitamin B$_3$ and vitamin C, became the centerpiece of orthomolecular psychiatry and continues to be so today.

Dr. Hoffer is editor-in-chief of the *Journal of Orthomolecular Medicine,* president of the Canadian Schizophrenia Foundation, and author of numerous books, including *How to Live with Schizophrenia, Vitamin B$_3$ and Schizophrenia,* and *Orthomolecular Medicine for Physicians.* In addition, he lectures internationally on orthomolecular medicine and has a private psychiatric practice in Victoria, British Columbia.

To date, Dr. Hoffer has treated more than 4,000 people with schizophrenia. "In my experience, going back now to 1955, schizophrenic patients on drugs alone don't get well. It's very rare. Even the strongest proponent of drug therapy will maintain that less than ten percent of these people ever go back to work. It's a very expensive disease. It destroys humanity; it destroys people. It's a

---

What Is Orthomolecular Medicine?

Orthomolecular medicine is the supplemental use of nutrients that naturally occur in the body (e.g., vitamins, minerals, amino acids, and enzymes) to rebalance an individual's disturbed biochemistry, that is, restore the molecular balance of the body. The application of orthomolecular medicine to promote mental health is known as orthomolecular psychiatry.

Nobel Prize-winner Linus Pauling, Ph.D., of vitamin-C therapy fame, gave this medical treatment approach its name in 1968. *Ortho* means "correct to normal." Orthomolecular medicine is based on the tenet of biochemical individuality, which holds that every individual's biochemistry is unique and treatment must identify and address the unique condition. Orthomolecular physicians also consider the effects of environmental and food supply toxins, and implement natural detoxification protocols as needed.

---

kind of living death because it strikes so early. It will strike a man who is 25, in the prime of his life, and he's finished. That is, if he is only given drugs."[171]

With orthomolecular medicine, one need not accept this dismal prognosis. A simple vitamin protocol results in a recovery rate of 90 percent in acute cases of schizophrenia, states Dr. Hoffer. He defines "acute" as patients with schizophrenia who have been sick for less than two years, who are having their first attack, or have recovered from the first and are having a subsequent attack. "With this group of schizophrenic patients, if they will cooperate with treatment for a minimum of two years, using the total approach, I expect about 90 percent to recover." This number is based on his clinical experience, the results of six double-blind controlled studies conducted by Dr. Hoffer and colleagues, and the results of other studies by orthomolecular physicians.

For patients to meet Dr. Hoffer's criteria for recovery, they must (1) be free of signs and symptoms; (2) get along well with their family; (3) get along well with their community; and (4) be paying income tax (or they would be paying income tax if they were being compensated for their work).

Among the chronic cases of schizophrenia, approximately 50 percent recover after ten years of orthomolecular treatment, says Dr. Hoffer, adding that not all will meet the fourth criteria for recovery, however. As schizophrenia often strikes in the late teens or early twenties, many of those who have been ill for years never got the chance to develop professionally or their illness left them with a poor work record that makes employers reluctant to hire them.

In Their Own Words

"I am certain of what has treated me. It is both the elimination of allergens plus the vitamins. . . . I am, for the first time since my preteens, relaxed, calm, stable and energetic. I am able to concentrate, converse and read without a 'second brain's' interference. I am no longer forced to rely on a day planner to remind me to eat, to bathe, to sleep, to rise."[172]
—A woman with schizophrenia, on her successful orthomolecular treatment

One of Dr. Hoffer's patients, for example, lost 13 jobs in a row due to his paranoia, aggressiveness, and hostility. With orthomolecular treatment, he recovered within two years and was then perfectly employable. Unfortunately, he could not get a job because of his employment record. "He is kind and considerate," reports Dr. Hoffer. "He gets along with his family, has friends in the community, travels a good deal, does volunteer work in nursing homes, but remains unemployed. He could have been working for the past eight years."[173]

In addition to saving and reclaiming lives considered lost, there is a cost benefit to orthomolecular medicine beyond the far less expensive price of treatment. For each patient who recovers, Dr. Hoffer saves the government $2 million, which is the estimated lifetime cost of care for a person with schizophrenia, whether untreated or treated with drugs.[174]

Dr. Hoffer concludes: "There can be no a priori reason why massive nicotinic acid [niacin] should not alter the outcome of schizophrenia. Apart from deep prejudice or sheer inertia, it is worth trying because it meets one of the major requirements of any treatment, that of 'doing the sick no harm.' Two-thirds of those who develop schizophrenia are more or less crippled by it

Dr. Hoffer defines "acute" as patients with schizophrenia who have been sick for less than two years, who are having their first attack, or have recovered from the first and are having a subsequent attack. "With this group of schizophrenic patients, if they will cooperate with treatment for a minimum of two years, using the total approach, I expect about 90 percent to recover."

and return to hospital for periods ranging from a few weeks to several years. Our studies suggest that at least half of the crippled two-thirds will be well if given nicotinic acid, and some of the others will be helped. We think that these young people, who are doomed to be in and out of mental hospitals for most of their lives, have a right to be given nicotinic acid even if medical people are skeptical. Nothing can be lost and as we have shown, belief or skepticism seems to have very little bearing upon the effects of this treatment."[175]

The Orthomolecular Model of Schizophrenia

"Schizophrenia is a syndrome, not a single disease,"[176] says Dr. Hoffer. "There are a whole variety of things that will mimic what we see as the final syndrome."[177]

This is precisely why natural medicine is well suited to the treatment of schizophrenia. A syndrome has no clear course of treatment because by conventional definition the cause is unknown; a syndrome merely describes a cluster of symptoms. Chronic fatigue syndrome is another example of these elusive conditions. Natural medicine surpasses conventional medicine in the treatment of syndromes because rather than focusing on a diagnostic label or the suppression of a cluster of symptoms, it focuses on the roots of illness, the underlying contributing factors that are combining to produce the manifesting condition.

Dr. Hoffer cites vitamin deficiencies and dependencies, mineral deficiencies, heavy metal toxicity, chronic infections, and allergies, among others, as things that can mimic schizophrenia. In his experience, food allergies, particularly to milk, wheat, and eggs, are a common causal factor. "They are really cerebral allergies, masquerading as schizophrenia or manic-depression."[178]

After encountering dramatic recoveries following the elimination of allergens, Dr. Hoffer more closely investigated allergies among his schizophrenic patients and found that of approximately 200 patients, "about 60 percent were allergic to foods and when these foods were eliminated, they improved or became normal."[179]

The allergy may not necessarily be to food. In one of Dr. Hoffer's patients, it was an allergy to aspirin that caused the schizophrenic syndrome. She had been routinely taking aspirin for hip pain. When she stopped, her schizophrenic symptoms disappeared and did not return.

The basic orthomolecular program for schizophrenia consists of dietary changes (a high-protein, low-carbohydrate diet and the elimination of white flour, refined sugar, food additives, and allergenic foods) and nutritional supplements, specifically, high doses of vitamin B_3 and vitamin C, zinc, and a B-complex formula to provide balanced B vitamins, with vitamin B_6, manganese, or other nutrients if indicated in individual cases.

Vitamin B_3 is the nutrient most implicated in the syndrome. "Schizophrenia could be classified as a B_3-dependency disease," states Dr. Hoffer. He uses the word dependency rather than deficiency because the vitamin B_3 requirement of schizophrenic individuals in order not to become ill is far greater than the usual amount that prevents deficiency.

"If you need, say, 20 mg of B_3 a day to prevent pellagra [a condition produced by niacin deficiency], if you eat a diet that contains 5 mg a day, you're going to get pellagra," he explains. "But suppose your needs are great, suppose you need 100 mg a day not to get sick. If you eat a diet that provides you with 20 mg a day,

The Basic Orthomolecular Regimen for Schizophrenia

Although individuals may require alterations and variations, the basic orthomolecular program for schizophrenia consists of elimination of "junk food" from the diet, which includes refined sugar, white flour, and food additives, avoidance of allergenic foods, and supplementation with the following nutrients:[180]

vitamin B_3 (niacin or niacinamide): 1.5 to 6 g daily, divided over 3 doses

vitamin C: 3 g or more daily

zinc gluconate or citrate: 50 mg daily

vitamin B-complex formula: once daily

If indicated on an individual basis:

vitamin B_6 (pyridoxine): 250 to 500 mg daily (frequently as important as B_3)

manganese: 15 to 30 mg daily (to offset tardive dyskinesia from tranquilizers)

omega-3 essential fatty acids: cold-water fish oil or flaxseed oil

you're still going to get sick. It's still pellagra, but it's now called a dependency. The problem is in your body and not in the diet."

Interestingly, both pellagra and scurvy produce schizophrenia-like symptoms. As noted, pellagra is due to a deficiency in vitamin B_3, while scurvy arises as the result of a vitamin C deficiency. These two nutrients are the primary ones in Dr. Hoffer's protocol for schizophrenia, although it was not their role in deficiency diseases, but rather their specific actions on adrenaline and a related substance, adrenochrome, that led to their central position in the protocol.

The Adrenochrome Connection

"Our theory, which I think is correct, is that there is abnormal production of one or more hallucinogens in the body . . . that act on the brain as if they had taken LSD," states Dr. Hoffer. "Their own body produces these hallucinogens and this is what makes them psychotic."[181] The hallucinogens, which arise from adrenaline, are adrenochrome and its relative, adrenolutin.

Adrenaline, released during the body's fight-or-flight stress response, is intended as a short-term mechanism for mobilizing the body in an emergency situation. It is highly toxic and must be rapidly converted into other substances

In Their Own Words

"My parents met me at the airport. . . .The first thing they thought was 'Uh, oh, chemicals, hallucinogenics.' That was what my sister and my brother thought, too, that I was taking a lot of LSD every day, because I was in that state every single day."[182]

—Ian, who reversed his
schizophrenia with
orthomolecular medicine

to avoid its damaging effects. "If I injected 2 mg of adrenaline into a person, I'd kill him because his blood pressure would explode," Dr. Hoffer explains. One of the body's conversion mechanisms results in adrenochrome, which becomes adrenolutin, as adrenochrome is too unstable to exist in the body.

According to the adrenochrome theory, people who are schizophrenic have a greater ability than other people to convert adrenaline to adrenochrome. This means that they are more exposed to its hallucinogenic properties, which are well established, says Dr. Hoffer. "When you give it to people, it, like LSD, makes them psychotic. Adrenolutin acts as a synaptic blocking agent, which is how LSD works."

Where vitamin B_3 comes into the equation is that it acts to decrease the production of adrenaline. As for vitamin C, high levels in the body help prevent the conversion of adrenaline into adrenochrome.[183]

As a preventive measure, it is advisable for people with schizophrenia to avoid factors that promote the release of adrenaline, with its attendant increase in adrenochrome. Stress, cigarette smoking, and food allergies are some of these factors. In regard to allergies, Dr. Hoffer notes that "one of the body's ways of dealing with a violent allergic reaction is to dump a lot of adrenaline into the body. If you go to the emergency room because you're having a reaction, they shoot you with adrenaline."[184] Thus, chronic food allergies result in increased adrenaline. Cigarette smoking not only promotes adrenaline release, but also depletes the body of ascorbic acid,[185] which makes adrenochrome conversion more likely.

Zinc Deficiency

Dr. Hoffer has found that zinc deficiency can also be a factor in schizophrenia, although it is not as common as vitamin-B problems. It tends to occur among people who have food allergies (an allergy to dairy or lactose intolerance is common), because the allergy interferes with absorption of nutrients, he says. Telltale signs of zinc deficiency are white spots on the fingernails, acne, sore knee joints, and severe PMS in women.

Another physician who has been practicing orthomolecular medicine for decades is Hugh D. Riordan, M.D., president of the Center for the Improvement of Human Functioning International in Wichita, Kansas, and author of *Medical Mavericks, Volumes I and II*. He gives an example of a schizophrenic patient for whom zinc was the answer: "We had a young lady who had been in the hospital for three months and was on sufficient psychotropic medication that she could not attend high school. She was one of those people who had white spots on her fingernails and painful knee joints. I started her on zinc and B_6, and over a couple of weeks she was able to get off her medications and was doing quite well. But as we've learned over the years, of course, no one really believes that anything could be that simple."[186]

Interestingly, with zinc deficiency, foods may taste bitter, which could help explain the paranoid belief previously common among schizophrenics that someone was trying to poison them. Dr. Hoffer notes that this used to be a much more common delusion, but is far less so today as the sweetness of most medicines has eliminated the association between poison and bitterness.[187]

For more about zinc, vitamin B$_6$, and schizophrenia, see chapter 4.

Saturation Point

Lack of biochemical measurement and lack of understanding of the concept of saturation point have contributed to the failure of the medical establishment to accept orthomolecular medicine, according to Dr. Riordan. The people who say that it does not work, he explains, are those who do not understand that it is necessary to evaluate the individual biochemistry to determine the specific nutrients that are most deficient in that particular person and then to saturate the system with those nutrients.

To take an example of a physical condition, "carpal tunnel syndrome is pretty well resolved when you have sufficient B$_6$ and other elements," he explains. "But you have to get to a 90 percent saturation. You can go from 50 to 70 percent saturation, but it does nothing for the symptoms. When you reach 90 percent, it's like a switch. You suddenly don't have any more problems." The length of time and the daily amount of nutrients it takes to reach the saturation point are not the same for everyone, however.

Dr. Riordan cites the case of one man in his twenties who had already been hospitalized three times for schizophrenic breakdowns. The biochemical picture obtained through blood and urine tests revealed that the nutrient he was most deficient in was vitamin C. He needed a very high daily dose (19 grams), and still didn't feel better until 11 months after starting the supplement protocol. At that point, he suddenly felt great. He had reached his saturation point, which flipped the switch on his symptoms. After that, he didn't need the high doses of vitamin C. He was able to cut down to two grams per day and remain well. His was not a typical case in terms of the dose required, but the point is that everyone is different.

"If a person is absorbing normally, most nutrients take one hundred days to saturate the system after one finds out what is missing," he states. As many people with schizophrenia are not absorbing well, reaching the saturation point, with its accompanying improvement in symptoms, tends to take longer.

"We view most chronic illnesses as sustained illnesses," Dr. Riordan says. "Chronic implies that it will never be cured. We see people as having sustained illness, and the question is if we can find out why the illness is being sustained." When it comes to schizophrenia or any other mental illness, the theme of ortho-molecular investigation is: "If your brain isn't working, look at how it's being fed, and what it needs to work better. The brain is the biggest user of energy in the body, and of course it's the first thing to go if you're not functioning well." Given these facts, Dr. Riordan is amazed that there is any questioning of the orthomolecular premise that nutrients are fundamental to mental disorders.

A Starved Brain

Michael Lesser, M.D., is cited by Dr. Hoffer as "one of the pioneers in the development of orthopsychiatry and medicine."[188] Practicing in Berkeley, California, he has 40 years of experience in treating schizophrenic patients (numbering in the thousands to date) with the orthomolecular approach. The author of *Nutrition and Vitamin Therapy* and *The Brain Chemistry Diet,* he has also published more than 50 peer-reviewed journal articles on ortho-molecular psychiatry.

Dr. Lesser regards malnutrition of the brain as the predomi-nant cause of schizophrenia, which is why orthomolecular treat-ment is the most helpful, in his experience. "We have to realize that if somebody screams or acts out of rage or does something psychiatrically bizarre, this is just the way that the brain has of expressing that it is starving, or being poisoned."

In the case of schizophrenia, Dr. Lesser has found that star-vation of nutrients, specifically those in the orthomolecular pro-tocol, is more the problem. As illustration of this, consider niacin. "The first noticeable symptoms of niacin deficiency are entirely psychological," he states. "Victims may feel fearful, apprehensive, suspicious, and worry excessively with a gloomy, downcast, angry, and depressed outlook."[189]

As noted previously, schizophrenics may require far more of certain nutrients in order not to suffer deficiency. For example, one study found that schizophrenic subjects required ten times the dose of vitamin C compared to a control group in order for traces of vitamin C to show in urine samples.[190] Traces in the urine indicate that the body has reached its saturation point; thus those with schizophrenia required far more vitamin C to reach that point.

Due to the malnourished state of the brain in schizophrenia, a nutrient-rich diet is an important part of the orthomolecular protocol. The high-protein diet not only provides needed nutrients, but also increases the effectiveness of the niacin, says Dr. Lesser.[191]

In his practice, orthomolecular intervention produces improvement in 85 percent of his patients. Most of the people who come to him are the chronically schizophrenic, rather than the acute cases, for which the therapy is, in his experience, "even more successful." An 85 percent improvement rate for chronic schizophrenia is impressive. Dr. Lesser notes that orthomolecular treatment cures over time. "The longer a person has been ill, the longer it takes for them to get better."

In one case, in which the man had had a schizophrenic breakdown, which unfortunately entailed serious consequences, improvement began in only two months after starting the orthomolecular regimen. James, who was in his late twenties, had been ill for less than two years when he came to Dr. Lesser. The visit was prompted by a huge legal mess that had made James desperate for help. At the time his psychotic break occurred, he was a representative for a company that leased cars. He began to believe that the cars were his, made the leases out to himself, and drove around in the cars with his friends. The company pressed charges and James was facing a jail term when he sought Dr. Lesser's aid.

Two months after starting the standard regimen, he felt better and the improvements continued until he was fully recovered not long after. In his case, niacin was the crucial nutrient, recalls Dr. Lesser. James noticed when he took more niacin that he was more in control of this thinking. In jail for his criminal behavior, he continued taking the niacin, became an honor prisoner, and decided to go into the ministry.

In regard to the orthomolecular approach, Dr. Lesser emphasizes, "The treatment is unique in that it requires a lifestyle change, not just taking a drug. This requires a serious commitment from patients. They may have to change their diet and take a number of supplements for a long time. Though the results are good and commensurate with the effort, it does require an effort."

Weaning Off Psychiatric Drugs

Dr. Hoffer regards the use of psychiatric drugs as analogous to the use of a crutch for a broken leg—a temporary measure. "In the same way that one uses a crutch until a broken leg is healed, so one should consider the drugs as crutches to be used until the person is healed. Then the crutches can be discarded and only used occasionally."[192]

As the effect of the nutrients may take a while, given the severity of the deficit, psychiatric drugs are often a necessary adjunct, says Dr. Hoffer. Once the nutrient program has begun to take effect, he begins to wean the patient off the drugs. People with schizophrenia may need to take their supplements for the rest of their lives, although they may be able to lower the dosage. Orthomolecular therapy for schizophrenia is like diabetes treatment, in that it needs to be continuous, according to Dr. Hoffer. "As long as the therapeutic regimen is followed, they will remain well."[193] In acute cases, he advises his patients to stay on the protocol for at least five years after their recovery.

Getting off psychopharmaceuticals is an important step not only because of disturbing side effects and the fact that they do nothing to correct the underlying problem, but also because of a phenomenon Dr. Hoffer calls tranquilizer psychosis. This is the secondary psychosis that develops with long-term use of antipsychotic drugs. As patients' schizophrenic symptoms are decreased, the drug begins to act on them as it does on nonschizophrenic people—that is, it makes them psychotic. The symptoms of the drug-induced psychosis are not merely a return to their original psychosis, however. Tranquilizer psychosis is characterized by "apathy, inertia, dullness, impaired memory, impaired concentration, impaired judgment, and finally, inability to engage in productive employment."[194]

This is in sharp contrast to the orthomolecular protocol, which not only allows many people with schizophrenia to become contributing members of society, but also entails only a few harmless side effects. These are the flushing that attends niacin supplementation, potential nausea and vomiting with niacinamide, and potential diarrhea from the high doses of vitamin C. In rare instances, jaundice develops, but disappears with cessation of niacin supplementation.

Building the dosage of vitamin C slowly can avoid the diarrhea that occurs at the saturation point for the vitamin. The dosage below the amount that causes diarrhea is known as "bowel tolerance," which serves as a natural feedback mechanism to determine the proper dosage. If diarrhea does occur, simply lowering the dose removes the problem. If you are one of the people who experience nausea with niacinamide supplementation, lowering the dose or taking niacin instead is the solution.

As for the flushing, which is a sensation of heat and prickling that generally travels down the upper body from the head, it is harmless, typically only lasts a few minutes, and tends to become almost unnoticeable with ongoing supplementation. The flushing is the result of the vasodilation (opening of the blood vessels) produced by niacin. Dr. Hoffer observes that schizophrenics tend to flush less than other people. "Often they do not flush at all until they have started to recover. This is now the basis for a diagnostic test."[195]

Joseph: 40-Year Schizophrenia Reversed

Joseph,* 66, had been schizophrenic since he was 27 years old, when he had a breakdown that landed him on a psychiatric ward. He was hospitalized at least five times in the intervening years, during which he underwent five series of electroconvulsive therapy. He had not been able to work for the past ten years and

---

* This case study adapted, by permission of Abram Hoffer, M.D., Ph.D., from his book *Orthomolecular Treatment for Schizophrenia* (Los Angeles, Calif.: Keats Publishing, 1999): 37–39.

had become increasingly confused, to the point that he could no longer drive.

His schizophrenic symptoms included hearing voices and paranoid delusions. He believed that people were staring at him and plotting against him, and he repeatedly told his wife that the telephone was bugged. In addition to his confusion, his memory and concentration were impaired. He became agitated and excited at times.

When his wife and brother brought him to Dr. Hoffer, Joseph appeared retarded, was clearly confused, showed no emotional reaction, and gave only short answers to the questions put to him. At 250 pounds (his height was 5 feet 11 inches), he was also obese.

Dr. Hoffer learned that Joseph was on extremely high daily doses of chlorpromazine (Thorazine), lithium, and the tranquilizer perphenazine, and taking a drug to counteract the side effects of these drugs. He had Joseph take 1 gram each of niacin and vitamin C after each meal. In addition to its other benefits, the vitamin C would help reduce the toxic impact of the drugs on the body. Dr. Hoffer also had Joseph observe a sugar-free diet. Food allergies were not in evidence.

At the end of a month, he was already experiencing improvement and his family had reduced his Thorazine dosage. At the end of six months on the regimen, his Thorazine dosage was down to less than half the original amount, his perphenazine dosage had been cut in half, and he had lost 13 pounds. "His family members were pleased with his progress as they saw his pre-illness personality reemerging," recalls Dr. Hoffer.

Joseph had a setback when a severe bladder infection sent him to the hospital, where he was not allowed to take his vitamins. His condition deteriorated with every day that he was off his vitamins, and he was put on the antipsychotic Risperdal. When he was back home again, his family took him off the new drug and resumed the vitamins. Shortly after, Dr. Hoffer increased his niacin dosage to two grams after every meal.

A month later, Joseph had lost more weight, was walking more, was much less paranoid, and reported that the voices were receding. Dr. Hoffer reduced his Thorazine dosage again. Three months later, he could get through a whole day without hearing the voices. Vitamin E and folic acid were also part of his protocol now, the E to support the antioxidant activities of vitamin C, the folic acid because it improves the function of niacin.

Two years after beginning treatment, Joseph's schizophrenic symptoms were gone and he was off all medication. He no longer heard the voices, his memory had improved, he spoke easily, and his weight was down to 217 pounds. Two years later, he was still fine. "He fulfilled my criteria for recovery: he was symptom free and got on well with his family and with the community. I expected he would be back at his artist profession," says Dr. Hoffer. "He had reached my therapeutic objective: to get him off drugs, cured of his tranquilizer psychosis, and cured of his schizophrenia. The odds are very good that he will not relapse as long as he remains on his orthomolecular program."

Generally, the longer you have been ill, the longer it will take to recover, says Dr. Hoffer, but that is not always so, as the case of Joseph demonstrates. His recovery took only two years, despite the fact that he had suffered from schizophrenia for nearly 40 years.

The Evolutionary Aspect of Schizophrenia

While schizophrenia is a devastating illness, if untreated, there is a positive side to the disorder. Dr. Hoffer views schizophrenia as an evolutionary advance. "There's certainly no advantage to being schizophrenic, but there's a tremendous advantage in having the genes of schizophrenia without being sick," he says. First, in relation to the heightened ability to convert adrenaline to adrenochrome, a person with schizophrenic genes is better able to deal with stress than other people, notes Dr. Hoffer, adding the qualification that "this is when they are healthy because they don't have enough genes to make them schizophrenic or when they are healthy because of nutrition."

In general, schizophrenics are healthier than nonschizophrenics. They tend to age better, retaining their hair color longer and wrinkling less. They have a higher threshold of pain, can tolerate cold and privation better, and are not as susceptible to shock after a physical trauma.[196]

Perhaps most significant, schizophrenic genes appear to exert a protective influence against the development of certain diseases, notably rheumatoid arthritis and cancer. The incidence of these conditions among schizophrenics is far lower than among the nonschizophrenic population.

Schizophrenic genes appear to exert a protective influence against the development of certain diseases, notably rheumatoid arthritis and cancer. "If you are schizophrenic, your chances of getting cancer are very slim," states Dr. Hoffer. Of the more than 4,000 schizophrenic patients he has seen over the years, only nine of them had cancer and all nine recovered completely. In his nearly 50 years of practice, Dr. Hoffer has not had a single schizophrenic patient who died from cancer.

"If you are schizophrenic, your chances of getting cancer are very slim," states Dr. Hoffer. Of the more than 4,000 schizophrenic patients he has seen over the years, only nine of them had cancer and all nine recovered completely. In his nearly 50 years of practice, Dr. Hoffer has not had a single schizophrenic patient who died from cancer.

The explanation may lie with adrenochrome, which has a second property in addition to its hallucinogenic effects. Adrenochrome is a cell-mitotic poison, meaning that it prevents cell division (mitosis), says Dr. Hoffer. "If you have schizophrenia, it means you have too much adrenochrome, but that means you're not going to get cancer. If you don't have enough adrenochrome, you can't become schizophrenic, but you can get cancer."

This points to another evolutionary aspect of schizophrenia. Dr. Hoffer cites the major cancer epidemic facing humanity, with the incidence continuing to climb. "The survivors are going to be the patients with the schizophrenic genes," he says. "Eventually, our whole population is going to have the genes, but they will never be sick because we will be intelligent enough to make sure that every human has enough vitamins. If you give every person from the time they are born enough B_3 and maybe some of the other vitamins, in my opinion, schizophrenia will disappear."

> ## In Their Own Words
>
> *"I've spoken to a lot of parents who have gone the traditional route with their children because they're intimidated. . . . It took a lot of courage for me to actually look for another method because I was given such flak by the traditional medical profession."*[197]
> —Rosalie, mother of Darren, whose psychosis was reversed by orthomolecular medicine

Orthomolecular Medicine and Conventional Psychiatry

As is so often asked about natural medicine treatments, if the orthomolecular approach is so effective, why isn't it a standard part of conventional psychiatry? Dr. Hoffer cites a number of reasons for this, beginning with the tranquilizer model, which rules psychiatry, just as psychoanalytic theories did previously. "It's taken them about 30 years to recognize that Freud was wrong and that this is in fact a brain disease," says Dr. Hoffer.

"But even though they've recognized that it is a biochemical disease, they have no conception that if you're going to deal with a biochemical disease, you ought to restore biochemical brain function. And you can't do this with tranquilizers. With tranquilizers, you interfere with certain brain reactions, whereas with the orthomolecular treatment approach, you enhance certain reactions."

Another reason Dr. Hoffer cites for why orthomolecular treatments have not become standard practice is the three powerful foes that have long been ranged against it: the American Psychiatric Association (APA); government bodies such as the

NIMH; and the pharmaceutical companies. The effectiveness of the suppression of orthomolecular information need not involve a conspiracy among these three megaliths. With the drug companies, their focus is and always has been on doing whatever it takes to sell their products and maximize profit. "When treatment is determined by a bottom-line mentality, the only profit that flows from drugs is the long-term, unsuccessful treatment of the chronically ill," says Dr. Hoffer. "We cannot forget that the business of business is to make money, but the business of medicine is to cure the sick."[198]

With the APA and the NIMH, defending their current paradigm may be the operational factor. Anything that doesn't fit is given no notice or discredited. "The old paradigm was that schizophrenia was a very complicated psychosocial disease, which must have many multiple causes and which would take years of investigation and maybe decades of research before you'd have an answer," states Dr. Hoffer. "And we were claiming that schizophrenia was essentially a complicated illness, but with simple causes, in the same way that syphilis is very complicated until you discover that you can cure it by giving penicillin to knock off the bacteria. In other words, every disease in medicine is complicated until one discovers what to do about it."

As another example, Dr. Hoffer recalls how in the old medical textbooks, 30 or 40 pages would be devoted to how to deal with pneumonia, which was little understood at the time. Today, coverage of the illness requires little space in medical textbooks because the evidence is that standard pneumonia is easily treated.

So, in the early days of orthomolecular medicine, the medical establishment "couldn't conceive of the fact that something as simple as a vitamin or nutrition could be helpful for such a serious disease as schizophrenia was." Now, when schizophrenia is known to be a biochemical disorder, the APA/NIMH paradigm embraces tranquilizers as the answer and continues to maintain "that nutrition and vitamins have absolutely nothing to do with schizophrenia," Dr. Hoffer states. "The average doctor reads only about drugs. That's all they are taught. They take classes in pharmacology that teach about drugs. They don't take any classes in nutrition. They don't take any classes in the therapeutic advantage of vitamins."[199]

Interestingly, the psychological model died as hard a death as seems to await the tranquilizer model. The medical establishment held onto that paradigm and offered strong opposition to the advent of tranquilizers. "In fact it took a number of congressmen and senators to persuade the NIMH, which was run at that time by psychoanalysts, to give grants to study the tranquilizers," says Dr. Hoffer. There was likely a lot of drug company money behind this push for research, given the huge profits to be had in psychopharmaceuticals. As is most often the case with natural medicine, money is not poured into the study of substances such as niacin, which lack the moneymaking potential of drugs.

"Orthomolecular medicine is the treatment of choice for the schizophrenias," Dr. Hoffer states. "Any physician dealing with these patients and their families who does not advise them that this treatment is available, and the results obtained, is not enabling patients to make an informed consent to treatment."[200]

 For more information about orthomolecular medicine or to locate a practitioner, contact the International Society of Orthomolecular Medicine/Canadian Schizophrenia Foundation, 16 Florence Avenue, Toronto, Ontario M2N 1E9 Canada; tel: (416) 733-2117; website: www.orthomed.org.

4 Biochemical Treatment of Schizophrenia

William J. Walsh, Ph.D., specializes in the biochemical treatment of mental, emotional, and behavioral disorders. While biochemical therapy is essentially the same as orthomolecular medicine (see chapter 3), in that substances found naturally in the body are used to restore biochemical balance, it focuses on several different parameters in its approach to schizophrenia and other mental disorders.

Dr. Walsh is the heir apparent of the late Carl Pfeiffer, M.D., Ph.D., a pioneer in the biochemical treatment of illness, and of mental illnesses in particular. Before he died, Dr. Pfeiffer asked Dr. Walsh to establish a center to carry on the important work in which they had both been engaged for decades. The result was the Health Research Institute and Pfeiffer Treatment Center (HRI-PTC), a not-for-profit research and outpatient facility near Chicago, in Warrenville, Illinois. Designed as a collaboration between biochemists and medical doctors, HRI is the research wing and PTC the treatment wing. Dr. Walsh is the center's chief scientist.

Since its founding in 1989, PTC has treated approximately 3,000 people with schizophrenia, and 12,000 others suffering from bipolar disorder, depression and anxiety disorders, autism, attention deficit disorder, hyperactivity, and other behavioral, emotional, and learning problems.

"What I've been doing for the last 25 or 30 years," explains Dr. Walsh, "is trying to develop chemical classifications for conditions such as schizophrenia, bipolar disorder, depression, behavior disorders, and autism because every one of these terms is an umbrella term or a garbage term that encompasses different categories." The chemistry underlying the diagnosis is not only the key to individual treatment, but if biochemical commonalities could be found among individuals in each category, this could also potentially point the way to the cause of the disorder, with attendant prevention and even cure.

Looking at the illness biochemically is more meaningful medically and, in the case of schizophrenia, does not carry the stigma of the psychiatric label. "The patients call it the 'S' word," observes Dr. Walsh. "Really, what does it mean? It's a word given to a number of completely different conditions that require completely different treatment. It's a word that everybody finds demeaning and almost insulting. There's a degree of hopelessness to hearing that word. It's considered the cancer of mental health."

Identifying the specific biochemical imbalances underlying a person's schizophrenia takes the onus off the condition, provides specific direction and measures for treatment, and offers hope rather than hopelessness.

Although schizophrenia has a genetic component, that doesn't mean that the condition is "hopeless or incurable," says Dr. Walsh. "What genetics means, to me, is chemistry. Chemistry can be adjusted and corrected." He gives the example of someone with depression, in which a genetic component is involved (science acknowledges the role of genetics in depression). "Some people, whether with medication or with some other therapy, become free of depression. So does that mean it wasn't genetic? And they weren't really depressed?"

About 90 percent of the schizophrenic patients who come to PTC fall into one of three biochemical categories, while the remaining ten percent belong to what Dr. Walsh refers to as the "splinter types," the causality of which takes more investigative work to identify.

Symptomatically and biochemically, schizophrenia is close to bipolar disorder with psychotic features, states Dr. Walsh. "I've seen almost identical patients with identical symptoms and one is called schizophrenic and the other is called bipolar with psychotic features. I think it's just a matter of semantics." In addition, the blood and urine tests of people with the two conditions show the same results. "We can't tell the difference between the biochemistry of the schizophrenic and the bipolar with psychotic features."

In biochemical treatment, it is the details of the biochemistry rather than the diagnostic labels that provide the direction for therapy. This approach has the advantage of addressing each person's unique biochemical condition. In contrast to psychiatric drugs designed to elevate or lower one neurotransmitter or another, biochemical therapy gives the body only what it needs, and it does so safely. The problem with the pharmaceuticals is that they're "affecting probably five to 15 other neurotransmitters, altering these people's brains and causing these things called side effects," says Dr. Walsh. On the other hand, providing the body with missing nutrients, as biochemical treatment does, restores its innate ability to correct and regulate its neurotransmitter levels and function.

Biochemical Profiles of Schizophrenia

Biochemical imbalances can be mild, moderate, or severe, which has a bearing on whether a person develops schizophrenia or not. On the mild end of the spectrum, "if a person is in a great environment and life is pretty copacetic and calm, they may go through life without a breakdown," states Dr. Walsh. However, if a person on the mild end "has a nasty environment or some troubling traumatic events in their life, they might break down because of that. But at the other end of the spectrum, with severe versions of these imbalances, I think it's inevitable. It doesn't matter what their life circumstances are, it's going to happen."

While every individual is different, the three primary biochemical profiles found in schizophrenia are: overmethylation/ low histamine; undermethylation/high histamine; and pyroluria.

The Methylation Problem

In the 1970s Dr. Pfeiffer developed a biochemical treatment model for schizophrenia that forms the foundation for the approach PTC uses today with both schizophrenia and bipolar disorder. Dr. Pfeiffer's model was based on his discovery of high histamine levels in some schizophrenics. Others had low histamine levels. Histamine is an essential protein metabolite (a product of metabolism) found in all body tissues and, although most people associate it with allergies (it is what produces the runny nose, weepy eyes, and other signs of inflammation in an allergic reaction), in the brain histamine functions as a neurotransmitter.

Dr. Pfeiffer found that he could reverse or alleviate schizophrenic symptoms by giving supplements that normalized the histamine level, lowering or raising it as needed. He concluded from the effectiveness of this approach that histamine, as a neurotransmitter, might very well be the decisive factor in schizophrenia, recalls Dr. Walsh. "A lot of time has passed since his death, and there's a lot more evidence. It appears that histamine is actually a marker for methylation. People who are high histamine are undermethylated. People who are low histamine are overmethylated. What Pfeiffer did was accidentally stumble on the right treatment, on an effective treatment. He thought he was adjusting histamine, but what he was doing was adjusting the methyl-folate ratio."

Methyl is one of the more common organic chemicals in the body; methyl groups are present in most enzymes and proteins. Methylation is the process by which methyl groups are added to a compound, making methyl available for the many reactions for which it is needed in the body. Both methyl and histamine are major, ubiquitous chemicals in the body and they compete with each other, Dr. Walsh explains.

With too much methyl, the body overproduces the three neurotransmitters dopamine, norepinephrine, and serotonin. With too little methyl, the neurotransmitter levels are too low. Folates are the various forms that folic acid takes in the body. Folic acid, a member of the B-vitamin family, aids in the manufacture of brain neurotransmitters and thus needs to be available in the proper ratio with methyl.

On the basis of his research since the 1970s, Dr. Walsh now knows that the methylation factor operates not only in schizophrenia but in bipolar and other mental disorders as well. For example, high histamine and its attendant low methyl are also associated with obsessive-compulsive disorders. As with schizophrenia, most people with bipolar disorder have a methyl imbalance—either too much or too little. "The methylation factor highlights the importance of knowing what is happening in a person biochemically," observes Dr. Walsh. "For people who are overmethylated, taking drugs to raise neurotransmitter levels will be detrimental."

Overmethylation/Low Histamine

Also known as histapenia (low histamine), this is the primary biochemical pattern in 45 percent of schizophrenics, according to HRI-PTC data. This group tends to be diagnosed with paranoid schizophrenia. The overproduction of dopamine and norepinephrine, which is characteristic of overmethylation, has long been associated with paranoid schizophrenia, notes Dr. Walsh.

"If you look at the sequence, dopamine is converted to norepinephrine by an enzyme plus copper," he explains. "The recipe for paranoid schizophrenia is overmethylation, detected by low histamine, and the second factor is high copper. Virtually all of them have, for some genetic reason, a tendency for very high copper levels. So what that causes is dramatic imbalances in dopamine, norepinephrine, and high levels of adrenaline. These people are very active. It's like their adrenaline is always up. They can't calm down."

This is the type of schizophrenia identified by Dr. Hoffer in his adrenochrome model. Dr. Pfeiffer, who was a colleague and friend of Dr. Hoffer's, discovered ten years later that the illness labeled schizophrenia comprises at least three major diseases that are completely different, with the most common being the one Hoffer found. The other two are the pyroluric schizophrenics and those with high histamine rather than low histamine.

Paranoid schizophrenia afflicts more women than men, which has to do with the relationship between hormones and the high copper associated with this form of the illness, says Dr. Walsh. The more estrogen one has, the more copper one has. (See Pyroluria for more about the role of copper in schizophrenia.)

With overmethylated schizophrenics, the primary psychotic symptom is auditory hallucinations. "It's usually a male voice, condemning them and telling them to do terrible things. They either think it's the voice of the devil or the voice of God. I must have heard that two thousand times," says Dr. Walsh.

In illustrating how the voices can begin and progress to psychosis, he gives an example of a 22-year-old man who was driving home from work one day and heard a voice calling his name in the car. He thought there was someone in the back who was going to rob him. He drove to a police station and got a policeman. They searched the car and looked in the trunk, but there was nobody there. The young man proceeded home and heard the voice again. This time he thought that one of the wise guys at work must be playing a trick on him by planting a little speaker in his car. When he got home, he searched the car for the microphone, but again didn't find anything. Over the next few days, he started hearing voices everywhere and all the time. They came out of his television and radio, even when they weren't turned on. "These voices beat at you day after day, week after week, and eventually they wear you down and overwhelm you," Dr. Walsh observes.

Other symptoms characteristic of histapenia are suicidal depression, religiosity, and problems with sleep.[201]

Symptoms can often be eliminated with biochemical treatment, which consists of supplements to reduce methyl, notably folic acid, vitamin B_{12}, and vitamin B_3 (niacin or niacinamide). Many people in the overmethylation category also have a metal metabolism problem, as evidenced by their high levels of copper in relationship to low zinc, so that problem needs to be addressed as well (see the section on metal metabolism to follow). It typically takes six to eight months of treatment for people to reach the degree of recovery that will occur in their individual case.

Undermethylation/High Histamine

Called histadelia (high histamine), this biochemical pattern is the primary one present in 18 percent of schizophrenics. Those having this pattern tend to receive a diagnosis of schizoaffective disorder, delusional disorder, or catatonic schizophrenia.

Their psychosis tends to be characterized by a thought disorder rather than a sensory disorder, such as the auditory hallucinations common among low-histamine schizophrenics. Typically, the dominant symptom is delusionary thought. However, "they usually seem quite calm; in fact, they almost seem catatonic," says Dr. Walsh. "It may be hard to pull words out of them and engage them in conversation. Almost all catatonic-type schizophrenics are high-histamine, undermethylated people. I think it has a lot to do with the fact that they have so little adrenaline."

Some people with this biochemistry may seem quite normal, until you encounter the delusion, which is often the belief that they are being followed by the FBI or the CIA. Obsessive-compulsiveness, characterized by the necessity to observe certain proscribed rituals and do things in the same way every day, may also be present. Seasonal allergies are also associated with high histamine, as are severe depression and blank-mindedness.[202]

The supplements used in treating high histamine and undermethylation are the amino acid methionine, calcium, magnesium, and vitamin B_6. These supplements increase methyl in the body and/or assist in methylation. Calcium is an important supplement for those who are undermethylated because it helps lower histamine levels. For those people who do not efficiently convert methionine to SAMe (S-adenosyl methionine), a necessary step in making methyl available to the body, SAMe supplements are part of their program.

With this protocol, "neurotransmitter production will become more normal," Dr. Walsh explains. However, reversing undermethylation is "a slow, gradual process that takes four to six months to complete." For histadelics, 50 percent improvement after three months of treatment is common and it typically takes eight to 12 months for all of their psychotic symptoms to disappear.

In addition, the nature of high-histamine, undermethylated people sometimes interferes with treatment. It is important to

The High-Histamine Personality

There are many high-histamine people who are not schizophrenic. "What histamine does is it speeds up the body's metabolism," states Patrick Holford, founder of the Institute for Optimum Nutrition in London, England, which is devoted to furthering research into the connection between nutrition and health. "It 'turns up the fire.' [High-histamine people] tend to be compulsive and obsessive in their personality. They wake up early and their mind is always thinking. This is not a problem. There are an awful lot of very successful people, creative people, multimillionaires, and so on, and they are high-histamine people. They're kind of driven people. However, the high-histamine people tend to become deficient in nutrients because they burn nutrients faster. So if they're on a bad diet, that sort of obsessive tendency can flip over into mental illness."[203]

note here that this biochemical pattern exists not only among people with schizophrenia or other mental illness, but widely in the general population as well. Those who manifest schizophrenia have a more severe imbalance, genetic vulnerability, or other factors that combine to produce the disorder. "High-histamine, undermethylated people are intrinsically noncompliant," says Dr. Walsh. "High-histamine, undermethylated people are the kind of people who don't want to go see a doctor for anything. If they have a splitting headache, they won't even take an aspirin. They tend to be averse to treatment of any kind."

Pyroluria

In some cases of schizophrenia, tests reveal a condition called pyroluria, which is characterized by extreme deficiencies in zinc, vitamin B_6, and arachidonic acid, an omega-6 essential fatty acid. (These are the schizophrenics for whom Hoffer found that B_6 and zinc are the vital supplements in treatment.) This is the primary biochemical pattern found in 27 percent of schizophrenics.

A pyrrole is a basic chemical structure used in the manufacture of heme, which is what makes the blood red. Pyroluria is a genetic disorder in pyrrole chemistry, characterized by an over-production of kryptopyrroles (meaning "hidden pyrroles") during the synthesis of hemoglobin (the iron-rich component of the blood that carries oxygen). Since kryptopyrroles bind with vitamin B_6 and zinc, which are then excreted in the urine, this leads to deficiencies in these two nutrients. People with pyroluria may have low levels of the neurotransmitter serotonin, as vitamin B_6 is needed for its synthesis.[204] Also, GABA is a zinc-dependent neurotransmitter, so a zinc deficiency may have negative repercussions on this neurotransmitter as well.

The diagnoses typically given to pyrolurics are undifferentiated schizophrenia, bipolar disorder, or other "splinter" category. "It's really schizophrenia that they can't quite figure out," says Dr. Walsh.

"Pyrolurics live in a world of fear," he notes. "That's the thing that is the easiest to detect with them. They are frightened and fearful all the time. They're the people who can't bear to get on an airplane for fear it's going to crash. They won't go on a boat for fear it will sink. They're just constantly afraid." If the person has visual or tactile hallucinations, that also tends to indicate that the schizophrenia involves pyroluria. Finally, while stress plays a role in other types of schizophrenia, it is particularly a problem with pyrolurics. "With the pyrolurics, not only do they have a high-stress onset, but their relapses are almost always tied to stress."

The role of pyroluria in schizophrenia and bipolar disorder is consistent with the first breakdown typically taking place between the ages of 15 and 25. Dr. Walsh believes that puberty and the growth spurt of that time period exacerbate the biochemical imbalances by consuming zinc and elevating copper and thus trigger the mental disorders. "Hormones are related to copper," he explains. "The higher your estrogen level, the higher your copper level. Copper is related to paranoid schizophrenia, so that's a direct connection. Also, for the pyrolurics, zinc deficiency is a problem. When you go through a growth spurt, it consumes a lot of zinc, so a pyroluric under a growth spurt may become severely zinc deficient."

The classic signs of zinc and B_6 deficiency, which tend to go together, serve as an alert for pyroluria. These include sensitivity

Biochemical Profiles of Schizophrenia

Histapenia

Affects 45 percent of schizophrenics

Biochemistry: overmethylation, low histamine, high copper

Common diagnosis: paranoid schizophrenia

Primary symptoms: auditory hallucinations, paranoia, suicidal depression, religiosity, sleep disorders

Treatment: vitamin B_3, vitamin B_6, vitamin B_{12}, folic acid, zinc, manganese, vitamins E and C

Histadelia

Affects 18 percent of schizophrenics

Biochemistry: undermethylation, high histamine

Common diagnosis: schizoaffective disorder, delusional disorder, or catatonic schizophrenia

Primary symptoms: delusions, obsessive-compulsiveness, severe depression, blank-mindedness, seasonal allergies

Treatment: methionine, calcium, magnesium, and vitamin B_6

Pyroluria

Affects 27 percent of schizophrenics

Biochemistry: deficiencies in vitamin B_6, zinc, and arachidonic acid; high urinary kryptopyrroles

Common diagnosis: undifferentiated schizophrenia or bipolar disorder

Primary symptoms: fearfulness, visual or tactile hallucinations, severe depression, assaultive behavior, symptoms made worse by stress, sensitivity to light, poor wound healing, no dream recall, tendency to skip breakfast, preference for spicy food

Treatment: zinc and vitamin B_6

Splinter Types

10 percent of schizophrenics (4 percent gluten intolerance, 6 percent other splinter types)

Causes: gluten intolerance, cerebral allergies, thyroid deficiency, excessive water intake, essential fatty acid imbalance, and metal metabolism problems to light, little or no dream recall, a tendency to skip breakfast, and preference for spicy food. Pyroluric schizophrenics typically have light skin. Other manifestations of this disorder include severe depression, assaultive behavior, and poor wound healing.[205]

Treatment for pyroluria focuses on supplementation with zinc, vitamin B$_6$, and augmenting nutrients. Of the three primary patterns of schizophrenia, the pyroluric form responds the fastest and the most completely to biochemical treatment. Recovery is often achieved in two to three months. "These people suffer more than most people, but they're also the ones that are the quickest to recover," observes Dr. Walsh, adding that they are also the quickest to relapse if they stop taking their supplements.

Other Biochemical Factors

As stated earlier, 90 percent of schizophrenics fit into these biochemical classifications. The causes for the remaining ten percent "splinter types" are varied, and include gluten intolerance, cerebral allergies, thyroid deficiency, excessive water intake, essential fatty acid imbalance, and metal metabolism problems. Dr. Walsh notes that gluten intolerance can, all by itself, cause schizophrenia, and accounts for four percent of the splinter types.

Excessive water intake, which produces polyuria (not to be confused with pyroluria), excess urine output, is a factor for about one in every 300 schizophrenics, according to Dr. Walsh. The high water intake throws off their electrolyte and pH levels. "All you have to do is take their water away from them and they get better. It's quite rare, but you become alert to that sort of thing."

Essential Fatty Acid Imbalance

While in Dr. Walsh's experience, essential fatty acid (EFA) imbalances play a greater role in bipolar disorder than they do in schizophrenia, they can still be a factor. "Of the 300 major fats in neuronal tissue and the myelin sheath, four of them make up more than 90 percent of all this fatty material at brain synapses and receptors," states Dr. Walsh, adding that these fatty acids must be important to mental health.

The four fatty acids are EPA (eicosapentaenoic acid), DHA

(docosahexaenoic acid), AA (arachidonic acid), and DGLA (dihomo-gamma-linolenic acid). The first two are omega-3 essential fatty acids and the second two are omega-6s. As others have observed, the standard American diet, with its generally poor nutrition and emphasis on junk food, tends to result in an overload of omega-6 and a deficit of omega-3 EFAs, notes Dr. Walsh.

This imbalance is most often the one involved when an EFA factor is present in the undermethylated or overmethylated schizophrenic category. The therapy is omega-3 supplementation, specifically EPA and DHA, in addition to the rest of the biochemical protocol. Fish oil contains both, and is therefore a helpful form of supplement, but Dr. Walsh also uses products that are pure EPA and DHA. Flax oil does not work as well because it doesn't have a balance between EPA and DHA, and low EPA alone is not usually the case with people with schizophrenia, he says.

Essential fatty acids appear to be especially important for the pyrolurics, according to Dr. Walsh. The problem for them is not omega-3 deficiency, but rather, low levels of omega 6, specifically, arachidonic acid. In these cases, the EFA supplement needed is primrose oil or borage oil.

Testing essential fatty acids levels via bloodwork can determine if EFA imbalances are present and supplementation indicated.

Metal Metabolism Problem

A problem with metal metabolism (the regulation of metals, which include both necessary minerals and toxic heavy metals such as mercury) in the body can also be present in schizophrenia. Heavy metal toxicity is rarely the issue in schizophrenia, says Dr. Walsh. It is a matter of dysfunctional metal metabolism in relation to minerals, as evidenced by high levels of copper in relation to zinc, characteristic of the overmethylated form of schizophrenia. Undermethylated schizophrenics generally don't have metal metabolism problems.

High copper in relation to zinc indicates that the body is unable to control the mineral levels in the bloodstream. Normally, the body can maintain homeostasis (the proper ratio) of copper and zinc in the blood, regardless of diet or other factors, because this ratio is so crucial to many functions. This mechanism of homeostasis relies upon a vital protein called metallothionein; thus, an inability to maintain homeostasis indicates a metallothionein deficiency or malfunction.

Metallothionein is involved in many functions of the body, including immunity, brain and gastrointestinal tract maturation, and the regulation of metals. A deficiency in or inability to utilize this substance is associated with an impaired nervous system; mental difficulties; weakened immunity; and digestive problems including malabsorption, nutritional deficiencies, and the development of allergies.

Since there is no commercial test to measure metallothionein in the body, the Pfeiffer Treatment Center (PTC) relies on the ratio of blood levels of zinc, copper, and ceruloplasmin (a substance in the blood to which copper attaches) as indicators of malfunction of this protein. Treatment then consists of supplements to stimulate the function of metallothionein.

The PTC has long been expert at correcting disturbances in metal metabolism. "We've known for more than 25 years that two-thirds of people with behavior disorders have a metal metabolism problem," states Dr. Walsh. "And we've known for all that time that it was almost certainly a problem with metallothionein. The reason we were sure was because all of the metals that are managed by metallothionein are the very ones that are abnormal in these people."

For example, people with obsessive-compulsive disorder tend to have very low copper levels, he explains, as do sociopaths (people with antisocial personality disorder). Paranoid schizophrenics, on the other hand, tend to have extremely high copper levels. Dr. Walsh emphasizes that it is the *ratio* of copper to zinc that is important here. "We learned a while ago that you have to measure the ratio to get solid data. If you look at the individual elements, you can get fooled."

A metallothionein problem, which results in a failure to achieve homeostasis of copper and zinc in the bloodstream, is mainly a genetic disorder, according to Dr. Walsh. But a zinc deficiency (as is characteristic of pyroluria) can also create or further exacerbate the problem. "The primary nutrient needed in the formation of metallothionein is zinc, so if you're extraordinarily zinc deficient, that will disable the system," says Dr. Walsh.

In any case, biochemical treatment is the solution to reversing the problem. "Zinc, manganese, and vitamins E and C are all aimed at inducing and promoting normal functioning of metallothionein," explains Dr. Walsh, adding that selenium and glutathione (a relative of glutamic acid, an amino acid) are also very useful nutrients for this purpose. Vitamin B_6 is also part of the protocol because "B_6 and zinc work together, and B_6 is directly involved in the synthesis of some of the neurotransmitters."

Dr. Walsh has found this program to be quite effective. Typically, the copper and zinc level out and become normalized. "When the person achieves homeostasis of copper and zinc levels in the blood, you can conclude that metallothionein is operational," he says.

As the supplement program gradually brings the metallothionein protein into proper function, metallothionein detoxification work will resume. The emphasis here is on *gradual.* "We learned long ago that we don't dare suddenly bring it to life," Dr. Walsh explains. "Because if that happens, the metallothionein works so well that it suddenly causes an excessive amount of toxics in the tissues to be released all at once. And that could cause nasty symptoms and stress the kidneys." To prevent this, the dosages of the supplements that stimulate metallothionein are slowly increased over time.

Identifying Biochemical Imbalances

As part of gathering information for treatment design, Pfeiffer Treatment Center staff look "for the symptoms that tend to accompany the various biochemical imbalances that our work over decades has taught us are associated with these disorders," says Dr. Walsh. In the initial hour- to an hour-and-a-half intake, "we want to learn everything about that human being. We want to know their medical history, their symptoms, their personality, their life history, the kind of student they were, reaction to any medications they had. We want to know what happened at the time of their breakdown. We want to know what differences they felt and their family saw at the time of the breakdown. Did they shut down and become nearly catatonic, or did they become more physically active and talk constantly?"

This information gives clues as to which biochemical imbalance underlies the person's schizophrenia. Out of the three main biochemical profiles, there are actually five possibilities: one of the three by themselves, or pyroluria with either high histamine or low histamine. Dr. Walsh notes that, in the combination cases, it can be more difficult to get the complete biochemical picture. In cases where only one imbalance is present, the symptoms are clear enough that he usually knows which one is operational before the test results come back. The results almost always confirm his conclusions. For those who don't fall into the main classifications, further testing may be needed to determine the direction that treatment should take.

Blood and urine tests provide the confirmation of observation and the scientific basis for biochemical treatment. Blood tests are key in identifying undermethylation and overmethylation, urinalysis in identifying pyroluria. The information gained from these tests enables treatment to be tailored to the individual.

In addition to the Pfeiffer Treatment Center (see the listing for Dr. Walsh in appendix B), another clinic that specializes in this type of biochemical balancing is the Olive Garvey Center for Healing Arts at the Center for the Improvement of Human Functioning International (see the listing for Dr. Hugh Riordan in the appendix).

Restoring Biochemical Balance

While the supplements to correct the biochemical trends of schizophrenia tend to be the same, there is no standard protocol at the Pfeiffer Treatment Center. Treatment is based on individual biochemistry and dosage is determined according to a person's metabolic weight factor. This is a method of calculating dosages based on metabolism, Dr. Walsh explains. It is far more accurate than figuring dosage as a mere percentage of the standard 160-pound person. The latter method results in underdosing small people and overdosing big people. If you have someone who is 320 pounds, for example, it is not correct to give them twice the dose of a 160-pound person, says Dr. Walsh.

With the biochemical program, the results for schizophrenia are quite good. An HRI-PTC outcome study revealed that 20 percent experience a full recovery, with complete disappearance of psychosis; 65 percent have significant partial improvement; and 15 percent experience little or no improvement. Note that these numbers include all cases, both acute and chronic, and all of the biochemical and splinter types of schizophrenia.

PTC's success rate is "extremely high" with the pyrolurics and the low-histamine, overmethylated people, according to Dr. Walsh. "The toughest ones for us are the high-histamine, undermethylated people." Part of the problem with this group is compliance.

With the biochemical program, the results for schizophrenia are quite good. An HRI-PTC outcome study revealed that 20 percent experience a full recovery, with complete disappearance of psychosis; 65 percent have significant partial improvement; and 15 percent experience little or no improvement. These numbers include all cases, both acute and chronic.

In general, however, people with schizophrenia tend to be more compliant than people with bipolar disorder, for example. This may be because schizophrenics "suffer so dramatically," says Dr. Walsh. "Their pain is so enormous that they will do anything to get better. I think it's a matter of desperation for them." This is not to say that people with bipolar disorder are not suffering

In Their Own Words

"[Medication] relieves my mental stress, but I hate my bodily responses to it and the dulling of my healthy emotions. Therefore, I stop using the drug as soon as the storms in my mind subside. And I keep wondering why there isn't more emphasis on alternative therapies, such as the holistic programs used now by people with physical illnesses."[206]

—An artist, 37, who suffers from paranoid schizophrenia

greatly, but schizophrenics are further along the continuum of pain and dysfunction in life.

One reason for noncompliance may be negative experiences with medications. By the time most people come to PTC, they have been on many medications and suffered through their negative effects. In a not-uncommon occurrence, one young man recently told Dr. Walsh that he didn't think he could bear to live if he had to continue to take Zyprexa (an atypical antipsychotic) and Celexa (an SSRI). He was on a high dose of both and didn't think they were helping him. "He said he felt like he was a horse with blinders on and he could only see straight ahead when he was thinking about things," recalls Dr. Walsh. "It was an interesting way to describe the differences in his mental functioning. He would try to focus on something and would lose all perspective."

Compliance is an essential component of biochemical treatment because most people deteriorate rapidly when they stop taking their supplements. "You can correct schizophrenia, but you can't cure it," states Dr. Walsh. "Correcting it means that if they stay on the treatment, a lot of them are completely okay." In most cases, maintaining the biochemical balance requires ongoing supplementation. There are exceptions. "We have some patients who became completely well. Against our advice, they brought their medication level to zero and stopped our pills, stopped everything. A few of them are all right. Most of them tend to break down within six months, and usually faster than that."

The following case histories illustrate the three main biochemical profiles of schizophrenia, how biochemical treatment can reverse the condition, and how stopping the supplement protocol can lead to relapse.

Melissa: Low-Histamine, Overmethylated Schizophrenia

Melissa had her first psychotic break at the age of 20, when she was in college. Diagnosed with paranoid schizophrenia, her major symptoms were auditory hallucinations, paranoia, and anxiety. She also exhibited violent tendencies and would run away and dash in front of cars. Due to the severity of the breakdown and the possibility of Melissa harming herself or others, her family was unable to keep her at home and had to commit her to a state hospital.

There, she went through a variety of the old class of antipsychotics—Prolixin, Haldol, and Thorazine. These did little but sedate her, which made it possible to warehouse her, but did nothing to improve her condition. After she had been in the hospital for nine years, she was put on Zyprexa, one of the new atypical antipsychotics. On the new medication, she was no longer violent. Her family was thrilled by this development and brought her home.

When Melissa was 32, her parents brought her to Dr. Walsh. "Although the medication had eliminated her impulsivity and violent tendencies, she was a recluse in the house and still suffered from auditory hallucinations, paranoia, and anxiety. She didn't want to leave her room and would only come out and eat with the family for one or two meals a week. She would talk to no one, was hearing voices constantly, and was highly agitated and paranoid. She didn't want to go out and be with people because she thought they were giving her dirty looks and didn't like her."

Although she was well enough to live at home, her life was quite miserable and she had no socialization. She was on heavy medication, taking three different drugs. Later, as she began to respond to PTC treatment and her communication improved, Dr. Walsh learned that depression was part of her symptom landscape as well.

Melissa's histamine turned out to be so low that the laboratory tests couldn't even detect it. To address her overmethylation, Dr. Walsh gave her folic acid, vitamin B_{12}, and niacinamide with augmenting nutrients, including vitamins C, E, and B_6.

A month later, the voices Melissa heard were starting to go away and she was coming out of her room and talking to the family more frequently. When it came time for her three-month follow-up, to Dr. Walsh's surprise, Melissa drove to the appointment, with her mother in the passenger seat. This was great progress for her. In addition, she was now living around the house, instead of staying in her room, and she had called her old high school friends because she wanted to start seeing them. The voices were gone and her depression was reduced. "She still wasn't herself, but she was somewhat better," Dr. Walsh recalls.

The usual procedure at PTC is to see people once a year after their three-month follow-up to run the tests again and make any necessary adjustments in the treatment. A year later, Melissa again drove herself to the appointment, this time by herself. She reported that her symptoms were completely gone. She was off two of her medications and on one-third the dose of the remaining one, Zyprexa. With occasional mild depression her only complaint, she felt normal and now had a job.

Melissa kept her yearly appointments religiously and was also totally compliant with treatment, being careful not to miss taking her supplements. At her fifth year on the protocol, she was better than ever. She had a good career, was earning a lot of money, lived by herself in a nice apartment, owned her own car, and was independent. At the end of the appointment, she said to Dr. Walsh, "Before I leave, I want to tell you something. I've been sick a long time, and I got better a couple of times, but I always had a relapse. On this treatment, I've always felt that maybe I would have a relapse. I've always been afraid to have a relationship, because I didn't want to be a burden to somebody. Now, I know that I'm going to be okay for the rest of my life. I've met a man. I think we're going to get married."

That was four years ago. Melissa did get married, and she's fine. "She's one of those who I would consider completely better," observes Dr. Walsh. "She takes a little bit of medication, and she says she has no side effects because the dose is so low. Her doctor's not happy; he thinks the dose is too low to do any good. But I don't feel that way."

At another of her yearly visits, Melissa told Dr. Walsh that she doesn't talk about those 12 years of mental illness, which were more horrible than anyone can imagine. She compared it to someone coming back from war who doesn't want to talk about it. When Dr. Walsh suggested that perhaps she could write a book about her experience, she responded that she couldn't because the horrors were too great.

"One thing I've learned is that when people like that get better, life is more delicious for them than for normal people," he says. "We all take our mental health for granted. When you lose it and you know the torment, and then you're all right, you enjoy life more."

Ben: High-Histamine, Undermethylated Schizophrenia

Ben, 45, was an air traffic controller who had been suffering with schizophrenia from the age of 20. People at his workplace didn't know that he had a problem. Dr. Walsh has encountered among other patients this ability to hide their schizophrenia. He cites a paranoid schizophrenic policeman, who of course carried a gun, and a schizophrenic psychiatrist who was treating schizophrenics. Most schizophrenics are not able to hide it, however. The ones who can are usually the high-histamine type, according to Dr. Walsh. "They don't tell anybody about their delusions, and they look and seem quite normal."

Over his 25 years of illness, Ben cycled between severe and not severe states. Although he was on medication (Prozac and Risperdal), he still experienced severe debility once or twice a year. He had attempted suicide several times. His family—he was married and had children—had helped him through. When he came to Dr. Walsh, he was on a leave of absence from work. He had taken the leave because he felt that he wasn't mentally capable and he knew he had people's lives in his hands. He had been off work for six weeks and wanted to go back, but knew he needed help.

Ben was unable to concentrate for more than a few minutes. Anything longer than that was exhausting. For instance, he could read a few pages of a book, but he couldn't read a chapter. In addition, he was severely depressed and suffering from anxiety and panic attacks. He had become antisocial, avoiding people and parties, and preferring isolation.

Ben also had striking delusions. He thought that a neighbor was to blame for all of his problems. "A lot of these high-histamine people attribute all their problems to some person. It could be his wife, a neighbor, somebody at work. And if that person disappears, they will find someone else that will be the cause in their mind of what's gone wrong."

He had been diagnosed paranoid schizophrenic, but Dr. Walsh believes a more appropriate diagnosis would have been schizoaffective disorder. "The American Psychiatric Association studied the accuracy of mental diagnoses," he says. "They have not published the study; it's very secret. They wanted to find out how accurate were these diagnoses throughout the country. The story I heard from one of the psychiatrists involved in the study was that 40 percent was the error rate. The man who told me that smiled and said, 'Well, of course it's worse than that.' The labels are just labels, but even the labels are inaccurate and somewhat random."

In any case, Ben had the classic symptoms of schizoaffective disorder, including his tendency not to talk much, says Dr. Walsh. "He would just sit quietly and stare into space and you think nothing's going on. In part, it's an anxiety disorder where the anxiety doesn't show at all. Their minds are racing, but it looks like they're very calm and almost catatonic."

To correct the undermethylation, Dr. Walsh started Ben on methionine, calcium, magnesium, and vitamin B_6, with augmenting nutrients. After three months, he was about 50 percent better, which, as mentioned earlier, is a typical progression for histadelics under biochemical therapy. He was an atypical high-histamine person in that he complied with treatment, notes Dr.

Walsh. Meanwhile, Ben had returned to work as scheduled and continued to work throughout his treatment program.

At one year, he was completely recovered. Now, six years later, he is still free of psychosis and has been promoted at work. He is off the Prozac and on one-third of his original dose of Zyprexa. Dr. Walsh sees no reason to try to get him completely off the drug because he is on such a low dose that it is not causing any side effects.

Isabel: Pyroluric Schizophrenia

Isabel, 30, ran the family business. She kept the books, did all the hiring, and was the most capable person in her large family. When one of her sisters died suddenly, she had a mental break-down, exhibiting the classic symptoms of pyroluria. Suicidal, she tried to kill herself by jumping off a bridge, which resulted in broken legs. She was constantly afraid and highly agitated, "her mind going in 49 different directions."

It took the PTC staff three hours to get a urine sample from her because Isabel was so agitated, troubled, and indecisive. She would start, and then say, "No, I can't." The staff worked patiently with her until they got the sample, and the test results showed that she had severe pyroluria. "This made me happy," says Dr. Walsh, "because those people get better faster and more completely."

Isabel needed large amounts of zinc and vitamins B_6, C, and E. On this regimen, her condition began to improve in three weeks. At the two-month point, she was nearly her old self. After three months, she was completely recovered, and she returned to running the family business.

When she had come to Dr. Walsh, she had been on a number of medications. Feeling 100 percent better, she stopped taking the drugs and was still all right. "She was one of those who don't seem to need medication, which happens most often with the pyrolurics," Dr. Walsh comments.

Everything went fine for three years, at which point Dr. Walsh got a call from Isabel's brother, who reported that there was something wrong. Dr. Walsh told him to find out if Isabel had been taking her supplements. He called back with the information that she had stopped, probably two months before. "They don't relapse right away," Dr. Walsh explains. "Sometimes it's faster, sometimes slower." The family brought her to PTC again. She wasn't in as bad a shape as she had been the first time and in six weeks of being back on the supplements, she was normal again.

"She has now relapsed three times, each time because of non-compliance," reports Dr. Walsh. "I do not understand how any human being could be that horribly afflicted, find a rather simple, inexpensive solution, and then do it again." Isabel lives alone, and maybe that's part of the compliance problem. There is no one right there to help her stay on the protocol. She's been fine now for a year and a half, and Dr. Walsh hopes that she has learned that she needs to stay on the supplements.

Medication

As these cases illustrate, biochemical treatment makes it possible for many people with schizophrenia to discontinue psychiatric medications or significantly reduce the dose. Dr. Walsh reports that most who come to PTC are getting "a boatload of medications. The psychiatrists tend to go heavy. They don't want another breakdown, so they overdo it." The result is a lot of side effects that make taking the drugs anathema to some patients.

As the nutritional supplements correct the underlying problems, the person's medication needs diminish, often to the point of doses so low that there are no side effects, as was the case with Ben and Melissa. It is important, however, to reduce the medications gradually.

One of Dr. Walsh's severely schizophrenic patients suffered serious consequences when she didn't observe this proviso. A classic pyroluric, she was very suicidal and was on seven powerful medications to try to keep her from killing herself

When her family brought her to Dr. Walsh, he explained to her how the program was going to proceed, that she should stay on her medication while the biochemical treatment brought her back into balance. He told her that she would start getting better, feeling calmer, within about three weeks, and "then the fear would start to melt away, and the psychosis would disappear. At that point, she could expect to start feeling completely sedated and incredibly fatigued. I told her and her mother that when that happened, it's time to go out and celebrate, because that means she's getting better."

The sedation and fatigue are the effects those powerful medications would have on a nonschizophrenic person. The onset of these symptoms is not a signal, however, to throw away your medication. Dr. Walsh emphasized how important it is to work with a doctor to slowly reduce drug doses. Stopping the drugs quickly can plunge you back into psychosis.

It happened in just the way Dr. Walsh described. The symptoms melted away and the young woman was overjoyed. Unfortunately, despite his warnings, the woman felt so wonderful that she just stopped most of the medication. Within a week, she was slipping back into the same terrible state. Now she is working with the PTC psychiatrist, who is expert at devising medication protocols according to an individual's body chemistry, to gradually wean her off the medications. Dr. Walsh anticipates that she will be one of those who recover completely, but who will need to be on a low dose of one medication, "which is far better than a big dose of seven medications."

He reports that about a third of pyrolurics get off their medication. Some of them keep their medication on hand in the event that they undergo some dramatic stress, which tends to worsen their symptoms. In this way, they can take the medication as needed.

Histapenic schizphrenics are so prone to relapse that only five to ten percent are able to go off their medication. The same numbers hold for histadelic schizophrenics. The noncompliant personality trait characteristic of this group prompts many more to throw away their medication, but only five to ten percent are able to stay off it.

These percentages are higher among people from other countries, Dr. Walsh says. "If you look at the outcomes of schizophrenia in America versus Canada, Ireland, England, or Germany, you find that people who become schizophrenic everywhere else, even if they don't have treatment of any kind, don't tend to be as severe and as horribly afflicted. For some reason, schizophrenia in America is a more serious condition." The reason for this is unknown, but he wonders if the standard, nutritionally deficient American diet, high in processed foods and chemical additives, has something to do with it.

The Joy of Recovery

"Of all the things we do, there's nothing quite as thrilling as when a schizophrenic gets better," says Dr. Walsh. "It's wonderful when a child improves, or when a depressed person is no longer depressed, but there's something about schizophrenia—the joy when somebody becomes themselves again. It's the peak experience for everybody on our staff."

He tells of two people whose recovery particularly moved him. They were both young, with "extraordinarily severe" schizophrenia, "completely lost mentally." They met in the mental hospital, fell in love, and got married. They lived a marginal, poverty-stricken existence after that, both of them in and out of mental hospitals. Six years ago, they managed to seek treatment at PTC. Now, they're both working, they own their own apartment, and they haven't been in a hospital for six years. The psychosis is gone in both cases. "They're really quite inspirational," says Dr. Walsh. "They shared a tremendously bonding experience, they've been through so much together, and now they're dedicating their lives to helping other schizophrenics."

Having witnessed the reclamation of many lost lives, Dr. Walsh is frustrated that biochemical treatment is not standard practice in psychiatry. "I know there are millions who could be helped. And there are tens of thousands of medical doctors and psychiatrists who would love to be able to give this kind of benefit to their patients. They just don't know about it. We've been doing this work for quite a while. Carl Pfeiffer was doing this 25 years ago with great success. Hoffer's been doing it since 1955 with great success, and yet, no one will listen to us.

"The whole thing, I believe, is that in the Western world, everybody's trying to find a billion-dollar drug that will solve a problem—that's where the money is. There is very little effort, proportionately, going into understanding the basic mechanisms and molecular biology of schizophrenia. It's really a shame. The medical schools are all supported by drug companies. If you look at *JAMA [Journal of the American Medical Association]* and the *New England Journal of Medicine,* every other page is a big, beautiful advertisement from the pharmaceutical companies."

Dr. Walsh believes, however, that the effectiveness of biochemical treatment will eventually result in its widespread use. "It seems likely that the next century's treatments will implement natural body chemicals that restore the patient to a normal condition, rather than drugs that result in an abnormal condition," he states. "The world may eventually learn the wisdom of Pfeiffer's Law: For every drug that benefits a patient, there is a natural substance that can achieve the same effect."[207]

5 The Five Levels of Healing

While many people speak generally of the body-mind-spirit connection, Dietrich Klinghardt, M.D., Ph.D., based in Bellevue, Washington, has developed a detailed model that explains that connection in terms of Five Levels of Healing: the Physical Level, the Electromagnetic Level, the Mental Level, the Intuitive Level, and the Spiritual Level. The model provides a comprehensive way to understand and approach the treatment of any illness.

Dr. Klinghardt is internationally acclaimed for this brilliant model of healing and for developing a number of therapeutic techniques (see "About the Therapies and Techniques" at the end of this chapter) that have proven useful in the treatment of a range of conditions, including schizophrenia. He trains doctors around the world in both his model and the use of the therapies he developed.

While mental illness is not the focus of Dr. Klinghardt's practice, a psychiatric internship was part of his early medical training and he has treated more than a hundred people with schizophrenia since then, primarily in Germany, where he sees patients for part of each year. As more doctors are trained in his therapeutic approach, it is to be hoped that hidden causes of schizophrenia, such as the dental factors, allergies, viruses, and transgenerational energy legacies that Dr. Klinghardt has discovered in his practice, will become a standard route of investigation. The Five Levels of Healing model provides a map for this approach to treatment.

Health and illness are a reflection of the state of the five levels in a given individual. Schizophrenia, like any health problem, can originate on any of the levels. A basic principle of Dr. Klinghardt's paradigm is that an interference or imbalance on one level, if untreated, spreads upward or downward to the other levels. Thus schizophrenia can involve multiple levels, sometimes even all five, if the originating imbalance was not correctly addressed. Each of the contributing factors discussed in chapter 2 falls on one, or sometimes two, of the five levels. For example, viruses exert their effects on the Physical Level while heavy metal toxicity creates interference on both the Physical and Electromagnetic levels.

Another basic principle of Dr. Klinghardt's model is that healing interventions can be implemented at any of the levels. Unless upper-level imbalances are addressed, restoring balance at the lower levels will not produce long-lasting effects. This provides an answer to why rebalancing the biochemistry of the brain does not resolve some cases of schizophrenia. Treating the chemistry only addresses the Physical Level of illness and healing and leaves the causes at the Intuitive Level, for example, intact. The brain chemistry will soon be thrown off again by the downward cascade of this imbalance.

The Five Levels of Healing model also provides a useful framework for the natural medicine therapies covered in the rest of this book. You will see that they approach schizophrenia by identifying and treating disturbances at the different levels. In keeping with the holism of natural medicine, a number of the therapeutic modalities function on several levels (see chart, page 125).

The following sections describe the Five Levels of Healing in general and identify therapies that can remove interference at each level. Then we turn to a more specific discussion of the three levels that Dr. Klinghardt has found are most often the source of the problem in schizophrenia. Keep in mind that interference at different levels can manifest as the same condition in different people, so while the source of the problem for one person with schizophrenia or another disorder is on the first level, the source may be on the fourth level for another person with the same diagnosis.

The First Level: The Physical Body

The Physical Body includes all the functions on the physical plane, such as the structure and biochemistry of the body. Interference or imbalance at this level can result from an injury or anything that alters the structure, such as accidents, birth trauma, concussions, dental work, or surgery. "Surgery modulates the structure by creating adhesions in the bones and ligaments, which changes the way things act on the Physical Level," says Dr. Klinghardt.

Imbalance at the first level can also result from anything that alters the biochemistry such as poor diet, too much or too little of a nutrient in the diet or in nutritional supplements, or taking the wrong supplements for one's particular biochemistry. Organisms such as bacteria, viruses, and parasites can also change the host's biochemistry. "They all take over the host to some degree and change the host's behavior by modulating its biochemistry," Dr. Klinghardt explains.

"The whole world of toxicity also belongs in the biochemistry," he says. Toxic elements that can alter biochemistry include heavy metals such as mercury, insecticides, pesticides, and other environmental chemicals. Interestingly, heavy metals operate on both the Physical Level and the next level of healing, the Electromagnetic Level. Due to their metallic nature, they can alter the biochemistry by creating electromagnetic disturbances.

In addition, Dr. Klinghardt notes that even if the source of the problem is on the fourth (Intuitive) level, until you get the mercury out, therapies that operate on the fourth level won't be able to clear the interference. The mercury creates a kind of wall that prevents the other therapies from working.

All of these factors at the Physical Level—surgery, injury, dental work, nutritional imbalances, microorganisms, heavy metals and other toxins—can play a role in producing symptoms of mental illness, including schizophrenia, according to Dr. Klinghardt.

The therapeutic modalities that function at this level are those that address biochemical or structural aspects, from drug and hormone therapies to herbal medicine and nutritional supplements, as well as mechanical therapies such as chiropractic.

The Second Level: The Electromagnetic Body

The Electromagnetic Body is the body's energetic field. Dr. Klinghardt explains it in terms of the traffic of information in the nervous system. "Eighty percent of the messages go up to the brain [from the body], and 20 percent of the messages go down from the brain [to the body]. The nerve currents moving up and down generate a magnetic field that goes out into space, creating an electromagnetic field around the body that interacts with other fields." Acupuncture meridians (energy channels) and the chakra system are part of the Electromagnetic Body.

A chakra, which means "wheel" in Sanskrit, is an energy vortex or center in the nonphysical counterpart (energy field) of the body. There are seven major chakras positioned roughly from the base of the spine, with points along the spine, to the crown of the head. As with acupuncture meridians, when chakras are blocked, the free flow of energy in the body's field is impeded.

Biophysical stress is a source of disturbance at this level. Biophysical stress is electromagnetic interference from devices that have their own electromagnetic fields, such as electric wall outlets, televisions, microwaves, cell phones, cell phone towers, power lines, and radio stations. These interfere with the electromagnetic system in and around the body.

For example, if you sleep with your head near an electric outlet in the wall, the electromagnetic field from that outlet interferes with your own. An outlet may not even have to be involved. Simply sleeping with your head near a wall in which electric cables run can be sufficient to throw your field off. The brain's blood vessels typically contract in response to the man-made electromagnetic field, leading to decreased blood flow in the brain, says Dr. Klinghardt.

Geopathic stress, or electromagnetic emissions from the Earth, is another source of disturbance. Underground streams and geological fault lines are a source of these emissions. Again, proximity of your bed to one of these sources—for example, directly over a fault line—can throw your own electromagnetic field out of balance and produce a wide range of symptoms. Simply shifting the position of your bed in the room may remove the problem.

In addition, biophysical or geopathic stress amplifies the symptoms of heavy metal toxicity, says Dr. Klinghardt. Heavy metals are found mostly in the brain, where they work like antennas, he explains. They pick up the electromagnetic or geopathic interference, which exacerbates the symptoms of mental disorders. Repositioning the bed can eliminate this exacerbating effect.

Interference at the second level can cascade down to the Physical Level. The constriction of the blood vessels in the brain in response to biophysical or geopathic stress results in the blood carrying less oxygen and nutrients to the brain. The ensuing deficiencies are a biochemical disturbance, with obvious implications for brain function and mental health. If such deficiencies have their root at the Electromagnetic Level, however, it is important to know that you cannot fix them by taking certain supplements to correct the biochemistry, cautions Dr. Klinghardt.

For example, if an individual has a zinc deficiency, supplementing with zinc may correct the problem if it is merely a biochemical disturbance (a first-level issue). If the restriction of blood flow in the brain as a result of sleeping too close to an electrical outlet (a second-level issue) is behind the deficiency, taking zinc may seem to resolve the problem, but it will return when the person stops taking the supplement. Moving the bed away from the outlet will stop the electromagnetic interference and prevent the recurrence of a zinc deficiency.

Physical trauma or scars can also cause an electrical disruption, creating what is known as an interference field or energy focus. "If a scar crosses an acupuncture meridian, it completely alters the energy flow in the system," observes Dr. Klinghardt. An infected tooth or a root canal can accomplish the same. Dental interference fields are known as dental foci.

Heavy metal toxicity, from mercury dental fillings and/or environmental metals in the air, water, and food supply, can block the entire electromagnetic system. "We know that the ganglia [nerve bundles that are like relay stations for nerve impulses] can be disturbed by a number of things, but toxicity in general is often responsible for throwing off the electromagnetic impulses."

The therapies that address this level of healing are those that correct the distortions of the body's electromagnetic field. Acupuncture and Neural Therapy (see "About the Therapies and Techniques," at the end of the chapter) are two strong modalities for this level. Neural Therapy's injection of local anesthetic in the ganglion breaks up electromagnetic disturbances. You could call the local anesthetic "liquid electricity," says Dr. Klinghardt.

Another therapeutic modality that functions at the second level is Ayurvedic medicine (the traditional medicine of India). As it employs a combination of herbs and energetic interventions, it actually covers the first two levels of healing: the herbs work on the Physical Level, and the energetic aspect on the Electromagnetic Level.

The Third Level: The Mental Body

The third level is the Mental Level or the Mental Body, also known as the Thought Field. This is where your attitudes, beliefs, and early childhood experiences are. "This is the home of psychology," says Dr. Klinghardt. He explains that the Mental Body is outside the Physical Body, rather than housed in the brain. "Memory, thinking, and the mind are all phenomena outside the Physical Body; they are not happening in the brain. The Mental Body is an energetic field."

Disturbances at this level come from traumatic experiences, which can begin as early as conception. Early trauma, or an unresolved conflict situation, leaves faulty "circuitry" in the Mental Body, explains Dr. Klinghardt. For example, if at two years old, your parents divorced and your father was not allowed by law to see you, you may have formed the beliefs that your father didn't love you and that it was your fault your parents broke up because you are inherently bad. These damaging beliefs are faulty mental circuitry.

The brain replays traumatic experiences over and over, keeping constant stress signals running through the autonomic nervous system. These disturbances trickle down and affect the Electromagnetic Level of healing, changing nerve function by triggering the constriction of blood vessels, and in turn, affecting the biochemical level in the form of nutritional deficiency.

It may look like a biochemical disturbance, says Dr. Klinghardt, but the cause is much higher up. "Again, this is a situation you cannot treat with lasting results by giving someone supplements, Neural Therapy, or acupuncture." You have to address the third-level interference, the problem in the Mental Body.

Despite what people may conclude from the related names, so-called mental disorders aren't necessarily a function of disturbance in the Mental Body. The cause can be on any of the five levels, iterates Dr. Klinghardt. In fact, in most cases, the third level is not the source. In his experience, most "mental" disorders arise from disturbances on the fourth level. In all cases, the source level must be addressed or a long-term resolution will not be achieved.

Dr. Klinghardt uses Applied Psychoneurobiology, which he developed, to effect healing at the third level (see "About the Therapies and Techniques"). Among the other therapeutic modalities that work at this level are psychotherapy, hypnotherapy, and homeopathy.

The Fourth Level: The Intuitive Body

The fourth level is the Intuitive Body. Some people call it the Dream Body. Experience on this level includes dream states, trance states, and ecstasy, as well as states with a negative association such as nightmares, possession, and curses. The Intuitive Body is what depth psychologist Carl Jung called the collective unconscious. "On the fourth level, humans are deeply connected with each other and also with flora, fauna, and the global environment," says Dr. Klinghardt.

The fourth level is the realm of shamanism, the ancient tradition of spiritual or psychic healing (see chapter 9). Other healers who can work at this level to remove interference are those who practice transpersonal psychology. Stated simply, transpersonal refers to an acknowledgment of the phenomena of the fourth level, "the dimension where people are deeply affected by something that isn't of themselves, that is of somebody else. Transpersonal psychology is really a cover-up term for modern shamanism," observes Dr. Klinghardt, meaning that psychotherapists who acknowledge the importance of spiritual connection are facilitating the kind of healing that was traditionally the purview of shamans.

For healing of the Intuitive Body, Dr. Klinghardt uses what is known variously as Family Systems Therapy, Systemic Psychotherapy, or Family Constellation Work. Developed by German psychotherapist Bert Hellinger, the method addresses interference that comes from a previous generation in the family. In this type of interference, says Dr. Klinghardt, "the cause and effect are separated by several generations. It goes over time and space." Rather than a genetic inheritance of a physical weakness, it is an energetic legacy of an injustice with which the family never dealt.

 For more information about Family Systems Therapy and to locate a practitioner, visit the Bert Hellinger website at www.hellinger.com.

The range of specific issues that can be the source is vast, but it usually involves a family member who was excluded in a previous generation. When the other family members don't go through the deep process of grieving the excluded one, whether the exclusion results from separation, death, alienation, or ostracism, the psychic interference of that exclusion is passed on. Another common systemic factor involves identification with victims of a forebear.

"A member of the family two, three, or four generations later will atone for an injustice," without even knowing who the person involved was or what they did, explains Dr. Klinghardt. For example, a woman murders her husband and is never found out. She marries again and lives a long life. Three generations later, one of her great-grandchildren is born. To atone for the great-grandmother's murderous act, the child self-sacrifices by, for example, developing brain cancer at an early age, being abused or murdered, or starting to take drugs as a teenager and committing a slow suicide.

Systemic family therapy involves tracing the origins of current illness back to a previous generation. Sometimes an event is known in a family, sometimes it is not. By questioning a client, Dr. Klinghardt is usually able to discover an event from a previous generation that is a likely source of interference for the client's current condition.

"It's a form of self-punishment that anybody can see on the outside, but nobody understands what is wrong with this child—he had loving parents, good nutrition, went to a good school, and look what he's doing now; he's on drugs. But if you look back two or three generations, you'll see exactly why this child is self-sacrificing." Dr. Klinghardt notes that mental illness is "very often an outcome on the systemic level."

Systemic family therapy involves tracing the origins of current illness back to a previous generation. Sometimes an event is known in a family, sometimes it is not. By questioning a client, Dr. Klinghardt is usually able to discover an event from a previous generation that is a likely source of interference for the client's current condition. If no one knew about a certain event, such as the murder in this example, there are usually clues in a family that point to those people as a possible source.

For the therapy, the client or a close relative chooses audience members to represent the people in question. In our example, they would be the great-grandmother, great-grandfather, and the new husband. These people come together on a stage or central area.

They are not told the story, even when the story is known. "They just go up there not knowing anything, and suddenly feel all these feelings and have all these thoughts come up. . . . Very quickly, within a minute or two, they start feeling like the real people in life have felt, or are feeling in their death now, and start interacting with each other in bizarre ways," says Dr. Klinghardt.

> ## In Their Own Words
>
> *"I love life and want to live, to cry but cannot—I feel such a pain in my soul—a pain which frightens me. My soul is ill. My soul, not my mind. The doctors do not understand my illness."*[208]
>
> —Nijinsky, Russian dancer and choreographer, schizophrenic at age 29

The client typically does not participate, but simply observes. "The therapist does careful therapeutic interventions, but there's very little needed usually." The person put up for the murdered husband stands there, with no idea of what happened in the past, but then he falls to the floor. When someone asks, "What happened to you?" he answers, "I've been murdered." It just comes out of his mouth. Then the therapist asks if he wants to say anything to any of the other people. He speaks to his wife and it becomes clear that she was the one who murdered him. They speak back and forth, and "very quickly, there's deep healing that happens between the two," states Dr. Klinghardt. "Usually we relive the pain and the truth that was there. . . . It's very, very dramatic. . . . Then the therapist does some healing therapeutic intervention with those representatives."

Family Systems Therapy is not a long-term endeavor. Dr. Klinghardt has found that the releasing work can be completed rapidly, usually in one to three sessions. "The remarkable thing about the systemic work is that it is so quick," he says.

With removal of the interference that was transmitted down the generations, the client's condition is resolved, although the trickle-down effect to the lower levels of healing may need to be addressed. Often, however, healing at the higher level is sufficient. With balance restored at that level, the other levels are then able to correct themselves.

Dr. Klinghardt likens Family Systems Therapy to shamanic work in Africa, in which healing often has to be done from a distance through a representative because of the impracticability of a sick child, for example, traveling 200 miles from the village to see the medicine man. The representative holds a piece of clothing or hair from that child, and the shaman does the healing work on the stranger. "There's a magical effect broadcast back to the child," says Dr. Klinghardt. "The child often gets well. It's the same principle [with Family Systems Therapy]. We call it surrogate healing." He adds that Systemic Family Therapy has become very popular in Europe in the last two years, while it is still relatively new in the United States.

Dr. Klinghardt has developed a variation of this technique that enables the work to happen with just a practitioner and the patient in a regular treatment room. He accomplishes the same end without representatives of the antecedents, using Autonomic Response Testing (ART, a kind of muscle testing; see "About the Therapies and Techniques") to pinpoint what happened and engage in the dialogues that arise in this work.

He gives the example of a 45-year-old woman who had lived daily with asthma since she was two years old. Through ART, in a kind of process of elimination, Dr. Klinghardt learned that physical causes were not the source of the asthma and that it had to do with exclusion of some kind in a previous generation. Further exploration revealed that this woman's mother had lost a younger sibling when she was two years old. In this case, the woman knew of the event, but that was all she knew. ART confirmed the connection between this buried death and the asthma. Dr. Klinghardt stopped the session at this point, instructing his client to find out what she could about this family occurrence and then come back.

The woman's mother was still alive and told her that the baby died shortly after birth, was buried behind the house without a gravestone or other marker on the site, and was never mentioned again in the family. Everyone knew where the child was buried, but there was an unspoken agreement never to speak of her. Not only that, but the next child born was given the same name, as if the one who had died had never existed or, worse, had been replaced.

"This was a violation of a principle of what we know about Systemic Family Therapy, which is that each member that's born into a family has the same and equal right to belong to the family." Exclusion, even in memory, is a form of injustice, and creates interference energy that is transmitted through the generations. Exclusion of a family member in the past is frequently the source of disturbance at the Intuitive Level, according to Dr. Klinghardt.

The client came back for the second session, and Dr. Klinghardt put her into a light trance state. "In that trance state she was able to contact that being, the dead sibling, and say to her, 'I remember you now, I bring you back into my family, I give you a place in my heart, I will never forget you.' Then she cried, and it was a very transformative experience." He observes that this process required very little guidance from him and took only about 20 minutes.

During the session, the woman made a commitment to go back to the house where the child was buried—it was still a family property—and put a gravestone on her grave. After the session, the woman's asthma was clearly better. She rated it at 50 to 60 percent better, and reported later that it stayed that way. "It took her about three months to put up the gravestone, and she said the day after she set up the gravestone for that child, her asthma disappeared completely," relates Dr. Klinghardt. That was eight years ago and the asthma has not returned.

Dr. Klinghardt and others who practice Family Systems Therapy have seen similar connections in cases of mental illness, as you will see in the case of Sonya. Schizophrenia, bipolar disorder, chronic anxiety or depression, addiction, hyperactivity in children, aggressive behavior, and autism can all lead back to systemic family issues. In fact, Dr. Klinghardt estimates that "about 70 percent of mental disorders across the board go back to systemic family issues that need to be treated. People try to treat them psychologically, on the third level, and it cannot work. This is not the right level." Similarly, focusing on the biochemistry is not going to fix the problem when the source is at the fourth level.

The Fifth Level: The Spiritual

The fifth level is the direct relationship of the patient with God, or whatever name you choose for the divine. Interference in this relationship can be caused by early childhood experiences, past life traumas, or enlightenment experiences with a guru or other spiritual teacher. Of the latter, Dr. Klinghardt says, "Some enlightenment experiences actually turn out to be a block. If the experience occurred in context with a guru, the person may become unable to feel a connection with God without the guru. The very thing that showed them what to look for becomes an obstacle."

This level requires self-healing when there is separation or interference in a person's connection to the divine. Direct contact with nature is one way to reforge the connection. "True prayer and true meditation work on this level as ways of getting there, but it's a level where there is no possibility of interaction between the healer and the patient," states Dr. Klinghardt. "I always say, if anybody tries to be helpful on this level, run as fast as you can." He notes that gurus and other spiritual teachers belong on the fourth level and have a valuable place there, but have no business on the fifth level. If they trespass into that level, they are putting themselves where God should be, says Dr. Klinghardt. "It's very dangerous."

That said, a number of the therapies in this book clear impediments to spiritual connection at other levels, thus opening the way for individuals to reestablish balance for themselves on the fifth level.

Operating Principles of the Five Healing Levels

The levels affect each other differently, depending on whether the influence is traveling upward or downward. Both trauma and successful therapeutic intervention at the higher levels have a rapid and deeply penetrating effect on the lower levels, says Dr. Klinghardt. This means that both the cause and the cure at the upper levels spread downward quickly. For example, if a systemic family issue is strongly present at the fourth (Intuitive) level, it will have profound effects on the first three levels. Similarly, resolving that issue can produce rapid changes in the

Natural Medicine and the Five Levels of Healing

The chart below shows on what level the natural medicine therapeutic modalities in this book function.

Therapy	Level	Chapter
Applied Psychoneurobiology	Physical Body	5
	Electromagnetic Body	
	Mental Body	
Biochemical Therapy	Physical Body	4
Cranial Osteopathy	Physical Body	6
	Electromagnetic Body	
Family Systems Therapy	Intuitive Body	5
Homeopathy	Mental Body	7
NAET (allergy elimination)	Electromagnetic Body	5
Orthomolecular Medicine	Physical Body	3
Psychosomatic Medicine	Mental Body	8
Shamanic Healing	Intuitive Body	9

Physical, Electromagnetic, and Mental Bodies. The lower levels may correct on their own, without further remediation.

At the same time, trauma or therapeutic intervention at the lower levels has a very slow and little penetrating effect upwards. When you get a physical injury (the first level), for instance, it will gradually change your electromagnetic field (the second level), altering the energy flow in your body. It's a slow process, however. The same is true for healing. "If you want to heal an injury on the second level—let's say you have a chakra that's blocked—you can do that by giving herbs and vitamins (biochemical interventions) but it will take years," says Dr. Klinghardt. But if you do an intervention on the third or fourth level, it can correct the blocked chakra on the second level immediately, within seconds or minutes, he notes.

Schizophrenia and the Five Levels of Healing

As stated earlier, schizophrenia can be the result of interference or disturbance on any of the Five Levels of Healing. In his practice, Dr. Klinghardt has discovered that schizophrenia usually involves level one (Physical) or level four (Intuitive), with level four being the most common. Occasionally, level two (Electromagnetic) factors can be involved.

Dr. Klinghardt's approach is based on treating the underlying factors involved in illness. Many of the people with schizophrenia who came to him for treatment consulted him initially for other health problems. After treatment resolved the particular underlying factors present in each individual, psychiatric symptoms improved or disappeared, as did physical symptoms or conditions. In decades of using this approach to treatment, "it has been rare that a patient's psychiatric symptoms have not significantly improved or disappeared altogether," states Dr. Klinghardt.

Schizophrenia and the Physical Level

The factor on the Physical Level that is often present in schizophrenia, and bipolar disorder as well, is an underlying virus, says Dr. Klinghardt. The presence of a virus is determined through Autonomic Response Testing (see "About the Therapies and Techniques"). The viruses are typically contracted in the womb, transmitted from the mother to the fetus, and tend to be herpes viruses, such as genital herpes or herpes simplex (the virus that causes cold sores).

The mere presence of the virus in the body is not problematic in itself. It is when the virus is able to replicate that problems begin. In order to replicate, viral particles must be able to penetrate into new cells. Healthy cell membranes in the body prevent this from occurring. As cell membranes are made up of oils, such as essential fatty acids, the EFA deficiency characteristic of mental disorders has serious consequences. The compromised cell membranes in people with an EFA deficiency allow the viral load to rise.

This still may not be a problem until other factors combine to create an overload on the body's nervous and other systems that then manifests as schizophrenia or bipolar disorder. Dr. Klinghardt notes that the rapid hormonal changes of the teen years may be one of the factors that in combination with the virus serve to trigger these disorders, both of which typically have their onset in late adolescence or early adulthood.

Fortunately, says Dr. Klinghardt, it is a relatively simple matter to stabilize the system through supplementation with fish oil and coconut oil. The benefits of EFA supplementation (fish oil) in the treatment of mental disorders is thought to be due to the importance of EFAs in brain development, function, and health (see chapter 2). Another quality of EFAs may also explain their efficacy. They are powerful antivirals in that they strengthen cell membranes and in so doing suppress viral replication in the body. With underlying viruses common in schizophrenia, this antiviral activity has obvious application.

"After you've successfully suppressed the viral activity, the schizophrenia goes away or symptoms improve significantly in over half the cases," states Dr. Klinghardt, noting that these results are from the antiviral approach alone.

Changes in diet can address the viral issue as well, and are an integral part of Dr. Klinghardt's treatment approach. "With these dietary measures, schizophrenics do extremely well," he says. "They need to eat a diet that is not glycemic, which means a high-protein diet, with no starch, sugar, or grains." A glycemic diet promotes high blood sugar (glucose) levels. As insulin is needed for the breakdown of glucose, high glucose leads to increased production of insulin. The diet Dr. Klinghardt recommends prevents high blood sugar levels, which in turn keeps insulin secretion down. This is important because "insulin is one of the peptides that crack open the cells and make them leaky," meaning that their walls become permeable, he explains. Viruses can then enter the cells. Thus, higher insulin levels create an optimal environment for viral replication.

Other antivirals that Dr. Klinghardt uses are coconut oil, the South American herb uña de gato (cat's claw), and the herb cilantro. "We put almost everybody with schizophrenia on cilantro," he says. "It is a very strong antiviral compound." Cilantro is also a natural chelator (see "About the Therapies and Techniques"), meaning it gets heavy metals such as mercury out of the body, which has additional benefit for people with schizophrenia. "We usually try to cover three, four things with one intervention," he says.

Schizophrenia and the Electromagnetic Level

Heavy metal detoxification in itself has not shown as strong therapeutic results with schizophrenia as it has with other mental disorders, such as depression, for example. Nevertheless, "it is important with all psychiatric and neurological illnesses that people have a metal-free mouth," says Dr. Klinghardt, referring to mercury fillings and other metal-containing dental items.

As noted earlier, heavy metals can create interference on both the Physical Level and the Electromagnetic Level. The leaching of mercury from fillings, for example, is an ongoing source of exposure to a known neurotoxin, a Physical Level factor. "Probably the more important effect in terms of mental illness is that each metal has a strong electromagnetic field around it," notes Dr. Klinghardt. "The upper teeth are close to the brain. The field of metal crowns, metal fillings, and metal bridges impairs the blood flow inside the brain, and that's a very important thing with all the mental illnesses."

A word of caution is necessary regarding mercury filling removal, however. If it is not done correctly, it can be more harmful than leaving the fillings in. Removal needs to be done by a dentist who has been trained to do it safely and effectively, as mercury vapors and particles are released during the removal process. In addition, to complete the mercury detoxification, a chelation protocol (either oral or intravenous) needs to be implemented after the fillings have been replaced with non-mercury composite fillings. Chelation is a method for removing heavy metals from the body (see "About the Therapies and Techniques").

 For information about dental mercury, see the websites of: Dr. Joseph Mercola, at www.mercola.com, and Dental Amalgam Mercury Syndrome (DAMS), at www.dams.cc. For help in locating a dentist, call the DAMS National Office at 800-311-6265.

Schizophrenia and the Intuitive Level

On the fourth level, in the arena of family systems, Dr. Klinghardt has found that the pattern in schizophrenia is similar to that of bipolar disorder. The typical pattern in both is that the child identifies with more than one person from a previous generation. Or stated in another way, "the child is strongly identified with two completely different consciousness fields," explains Dr. Klinghardt. "One person was abused in a certain way and another one was excluded or abused in another way. There aren't enough offspring to take this on, and it all ends up in one person. That person develops two different streams of consciousness."

He gives the example of a grandfather who fought in Vietnam and participated in killing the children in a village. He also became involved with a Vietnamese woman, got her pregnant, and then abandoned her. Later, the man married and had only one child, who also had only one child, a son.

"Now, two generations later, there's one offspring, but two generations before there are two victims: the village children and the woman who was left with another child. The one offspring, the grandchild, has the job of atoning for both the massacre in the village and the illegitimate child that wasn't recognized, that wasn't nurtured. The grandchild will unconsciously be identified with the victims in the village, and behave like a child who has been murdered or crippled by machine-gun fire or agent orange or whatever it was. The child at the same time will behave as if it is an abandoned child whose father has disappeared. That split of being identified with two different consciousness fields at the same time in the same person, we very often find, is the cause of schizophrenia or bipolar disorder."

Through Family Systems Therapy, the dually identified person can make peace with the ancestors or victims and release the need to atone. As mentioned previously, this is not a long-term therapy, but can be accomplished in one to three sessions.

The following case illustrates how factors on three levels can contribute to schizophrenia and how undetected causes such as viruses and dental factors can be a source of psychotic symptoms.

Sonya: A Triad of Causes

Dr. Klinghardt first saw Sonya when she was 33. The symptoms for which she initially sought his help had come on gradually over the previous two or three years, and consisted at that time of fatigue, headaches, various body pains, mental fog, and memory problems. As you will see, her problems later developed into a psychosis that was diagnosed as schizophrenia.

Dr. Klinghardt determined that the problem lay with dental foci (as noted previously, an Electromagnetic Level problem). Several of her teeth were dead (meaning that the pulp, the live center of the tooth that contains cells, nerves, and blood vessels, was no longer functional) and there was infection in the surrounding jawbone.

Sonya, who lived in Germany, went to a dentist in Munich who, over the next two years, performed the major dental work she needed. He pulled the dead teeth, operated on her jaw to remove the infected pieces of jawbone, then installed bridges, two of which needed to be quite long to span two missing teeth. After the removal of the dental foci, her fatigue and other symptoms disappeared and she felt remarkably well. Unfortunately, she didn't get to enjoy her newfound health for long.

For the bridges, the dentist used a new material that contained zirconium, among other metals. Six weeks after her final dental session, during which he put in the last bridge, Sonya had a severe psychotic breakdown (the first of her life) with auditory hallucinations. Diagnosed schizophrenic, she was hospitalized and put on multiple antipsychotic drugs.

After six weeks, the doctors considered her stable and discharged her. Sonya went back to work. A few months later, when she tried to withdraw from the medications because of the side effects—dry mouth, dizziness, and nausea—she slipped into another psychotic episode and was rehospitalized, this time for four weeks. She consulted Dr. Klinghardt again after her discharge.

First, he found via ART that Sonya was allergic to the dental material used in her bridgework, particularly the zirconium. This was a disturbance on the Electromagnetic Level. "It was a bridge that doesn't tend to leak metals, so it wasn't toxic. But the metals had a certain electromagnetic field effect," said Dr. Klinghardt. As discussed in chapter 2, allergies can throw off the electromagnetic field of the body and those that produce mental symptoms are known as brain allergies. In Sonya's case, with the bridge situated in her head and her exposure constant, the situation was far more severe than occurs with intermittent exposure to an allergen.

Second, also through ART, he discovered that she had a viral infection in her brain (a Physical Level factor); in her case, it was a herpes virus. The herpes family of viruses are known to live in nerves and the central nervous system (brain and spinal cord), explains Dr. Klinghardt. "They were until recently thought to be 'silent' unless there is an acute outbreak, such as shingles [caused by the herpes zoster virus]. Now we know that, once a person is infected, there is constant low-grade activity affecting the brain, the nerves, and other tissues in devastating ways."

Dr. Klinghardt started Sonya on the antiviral protocol of omega-3 essential fatty acids derived from fish oil, one capsule containing 180 mg of EPA (eicosapentaenoic acid) and 120 mg of DHA (docosahexaenoic acid) four times a day.

He then used NAET, an allergy identification and elimination method (see "About the Therapies and Techniques"), to clear her of her sensitivity to zirconium and the other dental material in her bridge. NAET is based on the medical model of acupuncture, in which disease is diagnosed and treated as an energy imbalance in one or more of the body's meridians, or energy pathways. These meridians—there are 12 major ones—carry the body's vital energy, or *qi (chi)*, to organs and throughout the system. Acupuncturists rebalance a meridian's energy by treating acupoints, the points on the body's surface that correspond to that meridian, via the painless insertion of needles or the application of pressure.

According to Devi S. Nambudripad, M.D., D.C., L.Ac., Ph.D., who developed NAET, allergies create energy blockages in the body.[209] That is, the body's energy field regards the energy field of a substance—eaten, inhaled, or otherwise contacted—as incompatible with its own, and its presence disturbs the flow of energy along the body's meridians. One, several, or even all the meridians may be affected. The central nervous system records the energy disturbance and is then programmed to regard the substance as toxic. NAET uses chiropractic and acupuncture techniques to restore the smooth flow of energy along the meridians and reprogram the central nervous system to no longer regard the substance as incompatible energetically.

To clear an allergy, the person holds a vial of the offending substance while the NAET practitioner uses slight pressure, needles, or a chiropractic tool to treat the appropriate points to restore energy flow on the affected meridian(s). Keeping the vial in your energy field during this process reprograms the brain and nervous system to regard the substance as innocuous. In general, it is then necessary to avoid ingesting or otherwise having contact with the substance for 25 hours after treatment (24 hours is the time it takes for an energy cycle through all the meridians, with one hour added as an extra precaution).

Often, only one NAET treatment is required to clear an allergy. In Sonya's case, it took four treatments to clear the zirconium, which indicates that she was highly allergic to the substances and the resulting electromagnetic interference was severe. In some instances, problematic dental materials need to be removed in order to resolve symptoms. In Sonya's case, however, the NAET was effective and she was able to keep the zirconium bridges, which was fortunate because they were quite costly.

Dr. Klinghardt also used NAET to clear Sonya of her sensitivity to one of the antipsychotic drugs she was taking. They then undertook a slow withdrawal process from all of the drugs, which took ten weeks in all. During that time, Dr. Klinghardt repeated the NAET clearing several times, which lessened the effects of withdrawal.

On this program, Sonya was stabilized. A year and a half later, however, she had another psychotic episode, which told Dr. Klinghardt that there was something more to address. At that point, he turned to family systems exploration and uncovered an interference on the Intuitive Level.

When Sonya was five, her father, who was Italian, left the family. Her mother, who was German, became her sole parent and Sonya did not see her father again until a few years before she had her first psychotic episode. At that point, she wanted to reconnect with him, but felt no sense of connection when they got together. Instead, there was "a remarkable distance," which she found strange because she was ready to re-embrace her father. She was also struck by how physically different they were. She could see nothing of herself in him.

In a Family Systems Therapy session, Dr. Klinghardt set up a family constellation. He designated a person to represent her father and another to represent her, while Sonya watched. "It was very clear that the person representing her in the constellation didn't have any energy toward the father," he recalled. "So I put another man in—Mr. Unknown—as a representative of a possibility for a father. The representative for her immediately started crying, falling to the floor, wailing in tears of being touched deeply."

They ended the session and Dr. Klinghardt asked Sonya to gently and lovingly inquire of her mother if there was another man. When Sonya did, her mother broke down crying and admitted that she had had an affair with a French soldier at the time she was engaged to the Italian. It was completely unacceptable after the war for a German woman to be involved with a French man, while an Italian-German alliance was acceptable, so she went ahead with the marriage. She knew by the timing of the pregnancy that Sonya was the child of the French man, but she kept that secret until the day Sonya confronted her.

"When the truth was brought to light, there was a deep, deep healing in the family," says Dr. Klinghardt. As often happens in Family Systems Therapy, it took only one session to resolve the old issue that had been creating disturbance in Sonya, without her awareness. Healing required that she acknowledge her true father and restore him to his rightful place in the family. This can be done in the context of a therapy session and does not require an actual meeting between the people involved. After the healing of the family therapy work, however, Sonya wanted to track down her real father. She was able to do so, learned that she had sisters, and met other relatives, which brought further healing to the entire family.

It has been seven years since Sonya learned of her real lineage, and she has had no further psychotic episodes.

In summarizing this complex case, Dr. Klinghardt comments that the relief Sonya got (a year and a half free of psychosis) as a result of the correction of the dental foci and the viral issue was more than he would have expected given the strong Intuitive Level factor. The latter "was definitely the big piece, and until that was touched, the other treatment would not be enough," he says. "I'm not sure if we had just done the family work, without the viral issue, whether that would have succeeded. It really was a combination."

About the Therapies and Techniques

Applied Psychoneurobiology (APN): This therapeutic technique was developed by Dr. Klinghardt. Employing his muscle testing method (see ART, following) as a guide, APN uses stress signals in the autonomic nervous system to communicate with a patient's unconscious mind. "You can establish a code with the unconscious mind for yes and no in answer to questions," he explains. "The code is the strength or the weakness of a test muscle." APN can lead the way to the beliefs that underlie illness and exchange those beliefs with ones that promote balance in the Mental Body. This can produce dramatic shifts in the health and well-being of the person, notes Dr. Klinghardt.

Autonomic Response Testing (ART): ART, also called neural kinesiology, is a system of testing developed by Dr. Klinghardt. It employs a variety of methods, including muscle response testing and arm length testing, to measure changes in the autonomic nervous system. (The autonomic nervous system controls the automatic processes of the body such as respiration, heart rate, digestion, and response to stress.) ART is used to identify distress in the body and determine optimum treatment.

In general, a strong arm (or finger, depending on the kind of muscle testing) or an even arm length (in arm length testing) indicates that the system is not in distress. A weak muscle or uneven arm length indicates the presence of a factor that is causing stress to the client's organism.

Chelation: This is a therapy that removes heavy metals from the body, among other therapeutic functions. DMPS (2,3-dimer-captopropane-1-sulfonate) is a substance used as a chelating agent, which means that it binds with heavy metals, notably mercury, and is then excreted from the body. DMPS can be administered orally, intravenously, or intramuscularly. Other chelation agents are cilantro, chlorella, alpha lipoic acid, and glutathione.

NAET (Nambudripad's Allergy Elimination Techniques): NAET, developed by Devi S. Nambudripad, M.D., D.C., L.Ac., Ph.D., is a noninvasive and painless method for both identifying and eliminating allergies. It uses kinesiology's muscle response testing to identify allergies. Chiropractic and acupuncture techniques are then implemented to remove the energy blockages in the body that underlie allergies, and to reprogram the brain and nervous system not to respond allergically to previous problem substances. For more on NAET, see chapter 2.

Neural Therapy: Developed by German physicians in 1925, Neural Therapy employs the injection of local anesthetics such as procaine into specific sites in the body to clear interferences in the flow of electrical energy and restore proper nerve function. The interferences, or "interference fields," as they are known in the profession, can be the result of a scar, other old injury, physical trauma, or dental conditions such as root-canalled or impacted teeth, all of which have their own energy fields that can disrupt the body's normal energy flow.

Disruption in the body's energy field has far-flung effects, and can manifest in seemingly unrelated conditions. "Any part of the body that has been traumatized or ill—no matter where it is located—can become an interference field which may cause disturbance anywhere in the body," states Dr. Klinghardt.[210] Neural Therapy injections may be into glands, acupuncture points, or ganglia (nerve bundles that are like relay stations for nerve impulses), as well as scars or sites of trauma.

For more information about the therapies or to locate a practitioner near you, see the following:

APN, ART, and Neural Therapy: Dr. Klinghardt (see appendix B); websites: www.neuraltherapy.com and www.pnf.org/neural_kinesiology.html.

Chelation: The American College for Advancement in Medicine (ACAM), 23121 Verdugo Drive, Suite 204, Laguna Hills, CA 92653; fax: 949-455-9679; website: www.acam.org.

NAET: Devi S. Nambudripad, M.D., D.C., L.Ac., Ph.D., Pain Clinic, 6714 Beach Boulevard, Buena Park, CA 90621; tel: 714-523-8900; website: www.naet.com; also see her book *Say Good-Bye to Illness* (Delta Publishing, 1999).

6 Restoring the Tempo of Health: Cranial Osteopathy

Structural factors, specifically cranial compression and its far-reaching effects, may also be a component in schizophrenia. Cranial compression results from distortions in the skull caused by birth trauma or later trauma from injury, emotional stress, vaccinations, medications, or dental factors, such as mercury fillings or root canals, says Lina Garcia, D.D.S., D.M.D., of Schaumburg, Illinois, who specializes in holistic dentistry and cranial osteopathy.

Compression is constriction due to pressure exerted on a body part or system. The impact of cranial compression extends throughout the body, but the immediate effects in the head can be pressure on the brain and cranial nerves, with attendant compromise of neurotransmitter function and brain function in general.

Cranial distortions and compression can be corrected through cranial osteopathy. Dr. Garcia, who frequently works with psychiatric patients, many of whom are referred to her by their psychiatrists, has found that such correction can resolve some cases of schizophrenia, bipolar disorder, and severe clinical depression, among other conditions.

Dr. Garcia brings a powerful blend of therapeutic traditions to her osteopathic work. Her healing orientation began in her childhood in Brazil, when she discovered that she has what people call "healing hands," the ability to synchronize with the healing process and bring about positive changes in an ailment by placing her hands on the person's body. Practicality and family pressure resulted in her directing her healing talents into training in dentistry. She brought a holistic orientation to her work as a dentist, however, and became one of a growing number of dentists who understand the pervasive influence that problems of the teeth and jaw exert on the entire body.

 For more about the effects of dental factors, see chapter 5.

Dr. Garcia went on to train in cranial osteopathy and is a member of the Cranial Academy (a component society of the American Academy of Osteopathy). It is not uncommon for dentists to pursue osteopathic training after they learn that problems of the teeth and jaw often arise from distortions in the bones of the skull. She later returned to the energetic healing interest of her childhood and trained with numerous hands-on healers. She also trained with a clairvoyant (a person with psychic abilities) and later studied the Five Levels of Healing and Family Systems Therapy with Dr. Klinghardt (see chapter 5). Her work is now a potent blend of these disciplines.

Cranial Compression from Birth

While cranial distortion can occur through various traumas, a common source is birth trauma resulting from the use of an epidural and the drug Pitocin during childbirth.[211] An epidural block, or epidural for short, is a local anesthetic injected into the space around the lower spinal cord for pain relief during childbirth. Pitocin is the drug given to speed the contractions of labor and hurry the process along. The use of both is common in current obstetrical practice.

While they may be convenient for those involved, these substances can result in the baby's skull being subjected to incredible pressure during birth. Under normal conditions, the woman's pelvis reshapes itself to accommodate birth. This process begins long before the first labor contraction. When the baby drops in late pregnancy, that's already part of the pelvic reshaping. If you

What Is Cranial Osteopathy?

Osteopathy, or osteopathic medicine, began as a medical discipline in the late 1800s, introduced by physician Andrew Taylor and founded on the principle of treating the whole patient, rather than addressing symptoms on a crisis basis. The interrelationship of anatomy and physiology is central to osteopathy. Manipulation techniques have evolved as hands-on treatment for restoring free movement in the body.[212]

Cranial osteopathy, or osteopathy in the cranial field, was developed by William G. Sutherland, D.O., and is based on an anatomical and physiological understanding of the interrelationship between mechanisms in the skull (cranium) and the entire body.[213] The central component of this relationship is what Dr. Sutherland termed the *primary respiratory mechanism*, or PRM. This is "a palpable movement within the body that occurs in conjunction with the motion of the bones of the head."[214] The flow of cerebrospinal fluid (CSF), the fluid that bathes the brain and spinal cord, is integral to the PRM.

The cranial bones move rhythmically, alternating between expansion and contraction, and this motion is reflected in every cell of the body. Palpable means that the PRM can be felt anywhere in a patient's body by someone who is trained to feel it, that is, a person trained in cranial osteopathy. The PRM can be thought of as the intrinsic fluid drive in the system.

As treatment consists of restoring the full functioning of the PRM in the context of the whole body, it is not restricted to the sacrum, spinal cord, and cranium. Cranial osteopaths use gentle, hands-on manipulation and pressure to release areas of restricted motion. In addition to structural or pain problems, cranial osteopathy can be beneficial for conditions in virtually any system or area of the body, including behavior problems, seizures, developmental problems, allergies, asthma, frequent colds or sore throats, and irritable bowel syndrome, among many others.[215]

anesthetize the pelvis, as with an epidural injection, the reshaping that normally occurs is inhibited. When labor does not progress because the vital pelvic involvement has been turned off, Pitocin is introduced to force the uterus to contract artificially.

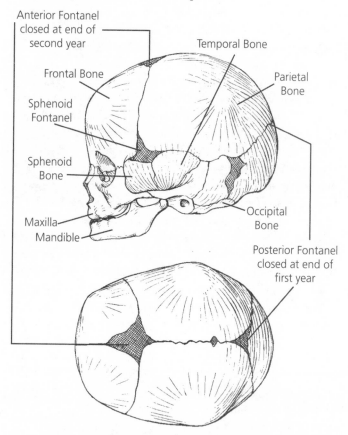

Anterior Fontanel
closed at end of
second year

Temporal Bone

Frontal Bone

Parietal
Bone

Sphenoid
Fontanel

Sphenoid
Bone

Maxilla

Mandible

Occipital
Bone

Posterior Fontanel
closed at end of
first year

Fontanels of Infant's Skull and the Main Bones of Skull

Osteopathic physician Lawrence Lavine, D.O., whose medical roots are in neurology and cranial osteopathy, among other disciplines, describes what follows as "using the child's head as a battering ram to force the pelvis to reshape to accommodate it. . . . Normally in labor, the head comes through, compresses, twists, then extends, and everything opens up. . . . When Pitocin and/or an epidural are used, distortions tend to be locked in."[216]

A newborn's head is made up of cartilage and membrane, except for two small areas of bone at the lower back of the head. There are two fontanels, or openings, in the membranous areas: the anterior fontanel in the front and the posterior fontanel in the back.

These openings and the fact that the cranium is not yet bone allow the sections of the skull to overlap so the head can get through the birth canal. Closed fontanels after birth indicate a misalignment of the cranial base, which is the base of the entire skull, where all the structures of the skull attach. If the cranial base is out of alignment, nothing that attaches to it can be in alignment.[217]

The result is compression on the brain, compression of cranial nerves, and systemic effects resulting from disturbance in the primary respiratory mechanism (see "What Is Cranial Osteopathy?"). Brain function can be compromised. In addition to the structural effects of compression on the brain, cranial compression may disturb neurotransmitter function.[218] Compression also diminishes cerebrospinal fluid flow, which affects all the other fluid systems of the body, including circulation. This leads to fewer nutrients and less oxygen being delivered to the brain.[219] Further, the compression in the skull makes the brain "irritable," and this irritability makes the brain far more vulnerable to adverse environmental influences, including toxins and stress.

The brain may be doubly irritated: first, by the compression on the brain from birth; and second, by brain allergies. The toxic effect of substances (food molecules) not normally found in the bloodstream (as occurs in leaky gut) and continual allergic reaction can irritate the brain as well. In addition, people can develop allergies to their own neurotransmitters. In this case, the body doesn't recognize its own serotonin, for example, instead regarding it as a foreign substance. The feedback mechanism sends the message that more serotonin is needed, so the body just keeps producing it, but the brain is unable to utilize it, which further compromises neurotransmitter function.[220]

See Also **For more about allergies, see chapters 2 and 5.**

Fortunately, cranial osteopathy releases the locked state of the skull, restoring it to its natural fluidity, thereby restoring the proper flow of cerebrospinal fluid and the function of the primary respiratory mechanism, removing structurally based interference in neurotransmitter and brain function, and returning balance to the body as a whole.

A case from Dr. Garcia's patient files illustrates how cranial factors and the separation of the Physical, Electromagnetic, and Spiritual Bodies (as explained by Dr. Klinghardt in chapter 5) can play a role in schizophrenia.

Darrell: TMJ and Schizophrenia

Darrell, 34, came to Dr. Garcia for treatment of TMJ (temporomandibular joint) syndrome, which involves misalignment of the teeth and jaw and can produce everything from headaches and neck or back pain to insomnia and depression, in addition to the more obvious jaw pain. TMJ problems are an indication that the bones of the skull are out of alignment, says Dr. Garcia. In Darrell's case, the TMJ syndrome manifested in jaw pain. Dr. Garcia used cranial osteopathy to realign the bones of his skull, which would in turn restore alignment to his jaw and teeth. Moving the bones allows the craniosacral system to "breathe" again, and "everything else breathes, too, including emotions," she explains.

Cranial osteopathy releases the locked state of the skull, restoring it to its natural fluidity, thereby restoring the proper flow of cerebrospinal fluid and the function of the primary respiratory mechanism, removing structurally based interference in neurotransmitter and brain function, and returning balance to the body as a whole.

All of a sudden, during this treatment, Darrell became "very dissociated." Dr. Garcia had already noticed in talking with Darrell that he was "one of those people who are not there." Treatment temporarily exacerbated his dissociation as it opened up his long-locked system. While the treatment was TMJ-oriented, Dr. Garcia never merely treats symptoms, so it was working at a deeper level to restore balance.

The next week, Darrell's TMJ problem was resolved, but he had a bad cold and was having a very hard time emotionally. In the week after a second treatment, his mental condition worsened and he was having trouble functioning at work. At his next appointment, Dr. Garcia looked at him and said, "Darrell, this is not the first time this has happened to you. If you want to talk about it, I'm here. Until you choose to do so, I can't help you."

After a delay, Darrell chose to tell Dr. Garcia his story. He had been hospitalized on a psychiatric ward and diagnosed with schizophrenia when he was in his early twenties. His mother was the only person in his life who knew. She had kept it from the rest of the family, and he had not told anyone about it until now. This episode was not his first. He had tried to commit suicide twice when he was younger.

What triggered the psychotic break that landed him in the hospital for a long stay was his involvement with a meditation institute and tutelage under a guru there. Darrell believed that the guru was using his mind, that he shifted something inside him "by looking into his eyes and changing something," which scared him. Between this and frequent meditation, the dissociation from which Darrell had been suffering since he was a child grew worse.

Dr. Garcia notes that while many people might dismiss Darrell's statement about the guru as the paranoia of a schizophrenic, in actuality, people who work with energy, as gurus do, can do a lot of damage if they are not working responsibly with the energy. People tend to accept that to work with people on the physical level, as in the medical profession, you need to be well trained. Working on the energetic level, however, is not generally subjected to the same standard. "But it is just as important to be well trained if you're working with energy," says Dr. Garcia, "otherwise it's the same as working in someone's mouth or on any part of them where blood is present without gloves and a mask." Without such protection, infection can pass between patient and practitioner.

For help in locating a cranial osteopath, contact the Cranial Academy, 8202 Clearvista Parkway #9D, Indianapolis, IN 46256; website: www.cranial academy.org.

The danger of transmitting energetic "pollution" is far greater because people are not educated in preventing it, as most medical personnel are in regard to transmission on the physical level. When someone is in a state of dissociation, those who work with that person on an energetic level have to be responsible about how they do it, Dr. Garcia cautions, for both their own safety and that of the patient. Otherwise, they may take in some of the energies themselves or introduce more foreign energies and cause the person to dissociate even more.

Some practitioners are simply not being careful or are not well trained enough, while others are well trained and step beyond the bounds of what they should be doing with a client, student, or patient, observes Dr. Garcia, which may have been the case with the master under whom Darrell studied. "I can't confirm this, but from an energetic point, it could easily have happened. You've got to be very careful where you go as a practitioner, and as a patient. It's far more serious than it looks."

During his involvement with the guru, Darrell's dissociation had increased to the point of a psychotic break. In the hospital, he was given shock treatment and put on medication, which he stopped taking not long after he was discharged. Since then, he had managed to keep himself together enough to work and to prevent people from learning of his disability.

The dissociation, in terms of Dr. Klinghardt's levels of healing, meant that Darrell's Physical Body was disconnected or dissociated from his Electromagnetic (Energy) Body and Spiritual Body. The result was the sense that "he was not present." Dr. Garcia notes that this disconnection is a factor in many of the psychiatric patients she sees.

"Their life force, their potency, their ignition system, as we call it, is depleted," she explains. "It's not being able to recharge itself. Every step of the way, everything is overwhelming. It takes too much out of the body to keep reigniting the system. The life force is not flowing. The body and the person are not working as a whole, but as separate parts. The physical, functional, energetic, and spiritual are disconnected."

Part of their overwhelmed state stems from the fact that their Energy Bodies are picking up so much information, according to Dr. Garcia. With the Energy Body dissociated

In Their Own Words

"My son has been a paranoid schizophrenic for nine years. . . . [I]n Jim's case . . . there was intrauterine complication, arduous birth, postbirth breathing block, and extreme colickiness. From what I have read it is possible that these factors might be implicated in some way."[221]
—Father, whose son became schizophrenic at 19

from the Physical Body, they have no boundaries and cannot differentiate the sources of information and what to do with them. "There are very different degrees of dissociation," she continues. "Some of us have a low degree where we can, by ourselves, without chemicals, come back. At the high degrees, you have schizophrenia." Healing involves reconnecting the Physical, Energy, and Spiritual bodies.

While numerous factors may contribute to the separation of the bodies, the success of osteopathic treatment does not depend on uncovering these causes. In some cases, the physical or spiritual body has been so much abused (by the various traumas mentioned earlier) that "the spirit decides to disconnect and have its own separate life," Dr. Garcia explains. One of the factors in Darrell's dissociation may have been his alienation from his family. His father had died when he was young and his mother physically and emotionally shut him out of the family. In combination with other factors, the result was the present state of disconnection between his bodies.

Osteopathic examination revealed that his cerebrospinal fluid (CSF) was not flowing well. The CSF has its own electromagnetic charge and when it is not flowing well, that charge is disturbed. This throws the Energy (Electromagnetic) Body, which is referred to in osteopathy as the individual's "potency," into a state of disorganization, Dr. Garcia explains. "If that is disorganized, it's the same as if your liver was extremely toxic, your kidneys were not eliminating properly, and your digestive system was totally overwhelmed."

To compensate for his depleted life force, Darrell had for years been pushing himself to keep going. "It was almost like having a superficial kind of ignition system," comments Dr. Garcia. The first osteopathic treatment opened him up a little, and he began to become aware of what had been going on in him. At that point, he fell apart, his immune system went down, and he got the severe cold. "Before, he was dissociated, but he was so used to it that he didn't notice. After I treated him, he had to take a step back before he could take a step forward. Before he could be present, he had to realize what he had been doing to survive."

Dr. Garcia's osteopathic focus with Darrell was to reorganize his potency (Electromagnetic Body). Bringing it back into an organized state would reconnect it to his Physical Body. For the first month, she treated Darrell once a week, and thereafter once a month. Her sessions last between half an hour and an hour, depending on the information she gets from the body and spirit of each person about what that individual needs at a particular time.

Part of the work was also to help Darrell to be comfortable with being present, feeling himself in his body. As he had been quite dissociated his whole life, living disconnected from his body, he at first experienced being present as scary and would seek refuge in dissociation without being aware of it. In a sense, he needed to be trained in what it was to be present and to recognize when he moved out of it. During treatment sessions, "every time he would go out of his body, I would say, 'You're out. You've got to come back,'" recalls Dr. Garcia. Doing the practical training in combination with the osteopathic treatment enabled him to shift relatively quickly.

Before he was able to accept the training in being present, however, he had to let go of the suspicious guardedness toward any practitioner that had resulted from his bad experience with the guru. "Once he trusted, and once he was aware of what was happening and was able to talk about it, things really shifted for him," said Dr. Garcia.

Darrell described his state prior to treatment as chronic, low-grade schizophrenia. He suffered from confusion along with his dissociation. He could maintain control as long as nothing too stressful happened in his life. When stress was added to his precarious state, it was too much for him to handle and could send him into an acute episode. And, if he wasn't treated properly, as happened with the guru, that could trigger another crisis.

While his condition worsened after his first osteopathic session as the treatment began the reorganization of his locked and restricted system, the worsening was only temporary. When his system was restored to its natural, balanced state, the result was restoration of health at all levels.

Without osteopathic treatment or another successful intervention, Darrell would eventually have had another breakdown, perhaps sooner rather than later, says Dr. Garcia. The signs were there in his life that he was reaching the breaking point. He wasn't sleeping well and was extremely fatigued. He was finding it more and more difficult to hold it together. He was getting confused and lost at work. "His appearance of functioning was a fake, not a true functioning."

To provide a strong nutritional base for his depleted system, Dr. Garcia recommended a low-carbohydrate diet and the avoidance of sugars. Darrell made these changes in his eating habits and felt so much better that "he doesn't want to go back. It has become a lifestyle change for him," she reports.

In Darrell's case, cranial osteopathy and dietary changes were sufficient to restore him to health. He didn't need the Family Systems Therapy that Dr. Garcia uses with some patients to explore transgenerational factors. It has now been three years since Darrell first came to Dr. Garcia, and he has not had another psychotic episode in that time. He recently moved to another state, has a new job, and is doing very well, truly functioning in work and other aspects of life.

Listening and Healing

Dr. Garcia's first step with patients is to talk with them about what's going on for them. What they say gives her information on both the Physical Level and the Electromagnetic (or energetic, spiritual) Level. Information about the Electromagnetic Level is not so much communicated to her through their words, but in what she picks up telepathically. She then does a hands-on osteopathic evaluation of the person's system, diagnosing how the cerebrospinal fluid is flowing, whether the potency in the system is strong or weak.

She describes her role in treatment as "listening to the information" that the body and spirit of the patient communicate if the practitioner is very still. "You don't dictate anything. You're not going in there and cracking bones and doing all of that," she explains. This is termed being an "efferent practitioner," which is a practitioner who waits to receive the information about how to proceed and what the patient needs rather than deciding where to work on a patient. It is the body and spirit of the patient that dictate the direction that treatment should take, and it is the gift of the doctor to allow this, she says.

Dr. Garcia's particular blend of healing disciplines and abilities makes what she does different from what most other osteopaths do. They have similar training, but her orientation is more to the electromagnetic, spiritual level of osteopathy, while theirs is to the physical level.

For example, in comparing her work with that of a close colleague, a physician who is also an osteopath, she notes that when they check a patient for diagnostic purposes, her tendency is to tap into the potency—the electromagnetic and the spiritual—while his tendency is to tap into the physical first. "He will go to the musculoskeletal and describe that well, whereas I will describe the electromagnetic and the spiritual in more detail," she notes. That's not to say that working on the physical level only is not healing, but Dr. Garcia seeks information from both body and spirit for the direction healing should take.

The information arrives silently and comes mostly from what osteopathy calls "the embryo." Osteopathic training involves extensive study in embryology, says Garcia, with the fundamental teaching that "in the first six to eight weeks of embryonic life, there's no genetic or environmental influences at all. The embryo has its own intelligence and is developing on its own." After that point, genetics and environmental factors begin to influence the developing fetus. Those factors comprise the first "lesion," as it is known in osteopathy, meaning "the first challenge that the embryo has to overcome." According to this model, if the mother is having a difficult time with her spouse, that emotional frequency will only influence the embryo after the first six to eight weeks, and not before.

The initial period in the life of the being, "when the embryo dictates the embryological development, when there is no other influence but its own intelligence and knowing," is the source of the body's wisdom. That is where the information comes from that the practitioner receives regarding how to restore the health of the system. It is "the pure intelligence of the body," which is later obscured and blurred by the toxins of external influences. Dr. Garcia regards this pure intelligence as part of the spirit.

Restoring health is like resetting the timing belt back to its original setting, that is, restoring the system's tempo to what it was in the embryonic stage before genetic and environmental influences intervened. "That tempo is health," says Dr. Garcia.

"I don't ever only treat the symptom," she notes. "I take the patient's whole body to neutral and go from there." Returning to neutral is the first step in restoring the system's natural, original tempo. Being in neutral means that the autonomic nervous system (ANS) is balanced, with neither the parasympathetic nor the sympathetic branch dominant. (The ANS controls the automatic processes of the body such as respiration, heart rate, digestion, and response to stress, with the sympathetic branch being the one involved in the high-adrenaline, fight-or-flight response to stress.)

With the ANS balanced, "the patient gets very calm and the whole system gets very quiet. Then when it's quiet, you've got to be very still as a practitioner, and wait for the health to dictate whatever else needs to be done in this system. It knows exactly what to do in different situations in the body. You're trying to balance the body by bringing that original self-healing ability back into focus. It's gotten so blurry."

It is necessary to synchronize with the health at different layers. Therefore, much of osteopathic work entails a purely musculoskeletal orientation, Dr. Garcia says. "Working on the body, you are unlocking the tightness, the rigidity, the obstacles that are keeping the cerebrospinal fluid from being able to flow optimally. Being a dentist, I really focus on the head; that's the cranial osteopathy. I check different parts of the body, but that's where I treat from."

In addition to birth trauma, any other trauma can lock up the system, according to Dr. Garcia. Any physical trauma, such as an accident or fall, emotional trauma, or spiritual trauma shocks the system. The spirit, for example, "may have been so tremendously abused that it's almost having its own life away from the physical," as mentioned in the case of Darrell. Spiritual trauma produces the same results as the physical trauma of a serious car accident.

Shock to the system causes it to lock up. It can stay that way for a whole lifetime, she notes. In the locked state, the system doesn't breathe or expand. "Every bone, everything in your system has to breathe, has to expand and contract to a certain extent. When bones are locked into one position, the system is not breathing enough. By moving the bones, by letting them breathe, everything else breathes, too, from the fluids to the emotions and spirit," Dr. Garcia explains.

Many people regard bone as hard, unshapeable, and immovable. On a practical level, this view is belied by what results from osteopathic treatment. Restoring the skull bones to their proper flexible position may produce noticeable structural changes or not, but a number of Dr. Garcia's TMJ patients say to her after treatment that their teeth come together in a different way than they did before—proof of bone movement.

When you consider the environment in which bones exist in the body, it is a vital milieu. The bones of the head and spine are bathed in cerebrospinal fluid. "Everything is surrounded by life, by liquid, by life force, by the electromagnetic," observes Dr. Garcia. "It's not a stagnant system at all." Regarding the body as purely musculoskeletal is "a very Newtonian perception and understanding of the system, of the body. When you go to Einstein and other wonderful scientists, you start seeing medicine in a totally different way. For example, in quantum physics, the quantum (the subatomic particle) is pure energy. It's an illusion that there's actually any physical to it. So medicine is the same. Some people, a lot of people, are still in the Newtonian knowledge and understanding of the mechanical existence."

The osteopathy that Dr. Garcia practices is a traditional model of osteopathy, in which the practitioner doesn't treat just the bone, but the fluids and the potency that are integral to the body's structure and which unlock everything from the physical to the spiritual. "Once you go deeper into treatments, the structure is just part of it." Restoring the body to its innate tempo (working as a whole rather than in disjointed parts), the state of balance and health that existed before genetics and environment intervened, allows the body, mind, and spirit to heal themselves. Given the genetic and environmental nature of schizophrenia, restoring the tempo of health in those who suffer from it can have far-reaching effects.

7 Rebalancing the Vital Force: Homeopathy

Homeopathy is what is known as an energy medicine, which means that homeopathic medicines do not contain biochemical components of the plants or other substances from which they are derived, but rather transfer their energetic patterns. The medicines help restore the individual's energy (vital force) to its natural equilibrium and thus return balance to the body, mind, and spirit. Disturbed energy flow is an underlying factor in any illness, including schizophrenia.

Judyth Reichenberg-Ullman, N.D., L.C.S.W., an internationally known naturopathic and homeopathic physician based in Edmonds, Washington, has seen the beneficial effects of homeopathic treatment for schizophrenia and other mental disorders. In fact, it was her interest in mental health and disillusionment with the results of conventional treatment that led her to homeopathy.

In her early career as a psychiatric social worker, she worked on a locked psychiatric ward, in emergency rooms, nursing homes, halfway houses, and patients' homes. "I saw the whole spectrum, and the suffering was terrible," she recalls. "I didn't see conventional medicine as having a magic bullet for most of these people. With the degree of side effects they were experiencing [from medications], I thought there must be a better answer."

Dr. Reichenberg-Ullman discovered that answer in homeopathy, as did her husband, Robert Ullman, N.D. They now teach, lecture, and have written numerous books together, including *Prozac Free: Homeopathic Alternatives to Conventional Drug Therapies.* Their column on homeopathic treatment has run in the popular journal *Townsend Letter for Doctors and Patients* since 1990.

They wrote *Prozac Free* to share their discovery of an effective alternative to medications for schizophrenia, bipolar disorder, depression, and other psychiatric disorders. "As shown by the numerous patients we have treated successfully, we believe we have found a method that can transform the lives of many people," she states.[222] "Certainly homeopathy can't help everybody, but the number of people that can be helped with these impairing mental and emotional conditions is incredibly gratifying."

Another homeopath, who is also a psychiatrist, has this to say about homeopathy's effectiveness in his foreword to *Prozac Free:* "In my 30 years as a psychiatrist I have found over and over again that nothing can match homeopathy in efficacy for treating mental and emotional illness when the provider of homeopathic treatment is a well-trained and competent classical homeopath," states Michael R. Glass, M.D., of Ithaca, New York. "Even in those cases where we cannot take the patient off psychiatric drugs, we usually can reduce the dosage and thereby decrease uncomfortable side effects, while at the same time producing real improvements in functioning."[223]

Homeopathy is safe, long-lasting, and has the further potential benefit of alleviating physical problems along with the mental/emotional symptoms for which someone with schizophrenia seeks treatment, says Dr. Reichenberg-Ullman. This is because homeopathy addresses the underlying imbalance that is responsible for all of a person's symptoms.

Homeopathy is safe, long-lasting, and has the further potential benefit of alleviating physical problems along with the mental/emotional symptoms[224] for which someone with schizophrenia seeks treatment, says Dr. Reichenberg-Ullman. This is because homeopathy addresses the underlying imbalance that is responsible for all of a person's symptoms. The imbalance occurs on an energetic level, which is why an energy medicine such as homeopathy is so effective in restoring balance. Let's look more closely at the concept of energy imbalance.

Schizophrenia and the Vital Force

We are energetic organisms, or energy-modulated organisms, explains Dr. Reichenberg-Ullman, and that energy is our vital force. "The vital force of each person, because of her makeup, has a certain susceptibility. Due to that susceptibility, there are going to be certain factors that trigger an imbalance or symptoms in that person."

For example, in a family with two parents who suffer from schizophrenia, which gives the children nearly a 40 percent chance of becoming schizophrenic, one child may develop the illness while others don't. That child was susceptible in some way. The same is true of nonpsychiatric illnesses, Dr. Reichenberg-Ullman points out, citing epidemics as an example. Even in virulent epidemics, there are people who are not susceptible and do not contract the illness, she notes.

Even with a susceptibility, or vulnerability, a triggering factor may not necessarily tip the balance into a psychotic breakdown unless the person's vital force is compromised. Traumatic events, stress, shock, illness, toxic exposure, and other life occurrences can compromise the vital force. In turn, a compromised vital force makes the person less able to handle future occurrences of this nature and the energy disturbance deepens.

"It's important to realize that the vital force, or the energetic equilibrium, of that individual is the bottom line," says Dr. Reichenberg-Ullman. "When there is an imbalance, a disturbance underneath the surface of the 'lake,' then there are ripples that go out. Those ripples can manifest in any number of ways. One of those ripples could end up being a biochemical imbalance, an imbalance in neurotransmitters, or a frank expression of a genetic tendency toward schizophrenia."

Scientific consensus currently holds that some problem with the brain's neurotransmitters is the factor behind schizophrenia, bipolar disorder, depression, and other mental illnesses. In actuality, the

research supporting this is "still more theoretical than they would make it out to be," says Dr. Reichenberg-Ullman. In her view, a deeper imbalance in a person's energetic equilibrium is what throws neurotransmitter supply and function out of balance.

Thus, simply attempting to correct the individual's biochemistry is not getting to the real source of the mental disorder. "You have to deal with that underlying disturbance, or else it's like putting your finger in the dike, which I think is what, to a large degree, conventional medicine is doing."

Like many natural medicine physicians, Dr. Reichenberg-Ullman regards symptoms, be they mental, emotional, or physical, as an individual's attempt to cope with the underlying disturbance. The body has its own wisdom, and symptoms are the ways in which a particular person adapts to the imbalance in its vital force. The beauty of homeopathy is that it goes to the heart of the matter and corrects the disturbance in the vital force. From that, all the other specific imbalances or symptoms correct as well. This is why homeopathy can address both your schizophrenia and whatever physical problems you are manifesting.

Standard laboratory tests have revealed the changes that transpire on the physical level, notes Dr. Reichenberg-Ullman. For example, she has seen cases of an overactive or underactive thyroid, as identified by tests that measure thyroid function, in which a second test taken after classical homeopathic treatment showed that the condition had reversed itself. She has seen similarly beneficial results in the red blood cell counts in people who prior to homeopathic treatment were anemic.

What Is Homeopathy?

To understand homeopathy, it is helpful to consider the derivation of the word as well as that of allopathy, both of which were coined by the father of homeopathy, Dr. Samuel Hahnemann, in the late 1700s. A German physician and chemist who became increasingly frustrated with conventional medical practice, Dr. Hahnemann devoted himself to developing a safer, more effective approach to medicine. The result was homeopathy, which arose out of his discovery that illness can be treated by giving the patient a dilution of a substance that produces symptoms resembling those of the illness, when given to a healthy person.

This principle, "let likes be cured with likes," became known as the Law of Similars. Dr. Hahnemann named this system of healing "homeopathy," a combination of the Greek *homoios* (similar) and *pathos* (suffering). At the same time, he dubbed conventional medicine "allopathy," which means "opposite suffering," to reflect that model's approach of treating illness by giving an antidote to the symptoms, a medicine that produces the opposite effect from what the patient is suffering. (A laxative for constipation is an illustration of the allopathic approach; it produces diarrhea.)[226]

A homeopathic remedy can be employed as a simple remedy to address a certain transitory ailment or as a constitutional remedy to address the more permanent constellation of physical, psychological, and emotional characteristics—the constitution—of an individual patient. A constitutional remedy works to restore balance and thus health on all levels.

Homeopathic remedies are prepared through a process of dilution of plant, mineral, or animal substances, which results in a "potentized" remedy, one that contains the energy imprint of the substance rather than its biochemical components. This is why homeopathy falls into the category of energy medicine; it works on an energetic level to effect change in all aspects of a person and restore balance to the whole.

Paradoxically, the higher the number of dilutions, the greater the potency and the effects of the remedy. (Note that the word "potency" as it is used here reflects the more traditional usage of the word, meaning "strong, powerful," as contrasted with the use of the word in osteopathic medicine, as discussed in chapter 6. Both usages refer to energy, however.) Thus, the higher the potency number, the more powerful the remedy. Remedies used to treat a transitory condition are usually 6C, 12C, or 30C, relatively low-potency remedies. A constitutional remedy is often a 200C potency, which means it has been diluted 200 times (99 parts alcohol or water to one part substance), or a 1M potency, which means it has been diluted a thousand times.

> ## The Benefits of Homeopathic Treatment
>
> Dr. Reichenberg-Ullman cites the following benefits of constitutional homeopathic treatment.[227] Homeopathy:
>
> treats the whole person
>
> treats the root of the problem
>
> treats each person as an individual
>
> uses natural, nontoxic medicines
>
> is considered safe and does not have the side effects of prescription drugs
>
> heals physical, mental, and emotional symptoms
>
> uses medicines, one dose of which works for months or years rather than hours
>
> uses inexpensive medicines
>
> is cost effective

Constitutional Treatment of Schizophrenia

Classical or constitutional homeopathic treatment is distinct from the use of homeopathic remedies for acute symptoms in that it employs a single remedy that addresses the particular and unique mental, emotional, and physical state of an individual. Dr. Reichenberg-Ullman explains it this way: "Each child, or adult, is much like a jigsaw puzzle. Once all of the pieces are assembled in their proper places, an image emerges that is distinct from other puzzles. It is the task of a homeopath to recognize that image and to match it to the corresponding image of one specific homeopathic medicine."[228]

The homeopath makes that match by considering the person's behaviors, feelings, attitudes, beliefs, likes, dislikes, physical symptoms, prenatal and birth history, family medical history, eating and sleeping patterns, and even dreams and fears.[229] By giving the remedy whose qualities match this unique cluster most closely, the homeopathic principle of "like cures like" is put into operation and the remedy works to restore the person to balance. People may have one constitutional remedy that is their match throughout their life, or it may change over time and a different constitutional remedy might then be required.

Homeopathy does not prescribe according to diagnostic labels, but rather according to the complete picture of the individual. Thus, there is no universal remedy for schizophrenia, and two people suffering from this condition will likely require two entirely different remedies, chosen from more than two thousand possible homeopathic remedies.

It's interesting to note that the qualities of the remedy that is the correct one for a person reflect their areas of susceptibility or vulnerability. "When a certain homeopathic medicine benefits a person, that tells me something about that person," observes Dr. Reichenberg-Ullman. "From understanding that homeopathic medicine, I know what kinds of conditions, whether mental, emotional, or physical, the person is likely to be susceptible to and what kinds they aren't. It often gives you a predictive capacity."

A single dose of a constitutional remedy is sometimes all that is needed at first (though the remedy may also be given more often, even daily). When the remedy is the correct one for an individual, changes can begin relatively quickly, within two to five weeks after taking the dose. (Some people experience changes in the first day, or even within hours.) If there are no changes within five weeks, that generally indicates that it is not the proper remedy. A remedy continues to work over time, anywhere from four months to a year or longer. Repeat doses may be necessary if there is a relapse of symptoms, or sometimes a different remedy may be called for.

Due to the way homeopathic remedies work, it is important to continue treatment for at least two years, and in the case of schizophrenia, usually five years or longer, states Dr. Reichenberg-Ullman. This does not necessarily entail frequent appointments with your homeopath, however. As stated, a single dose of a remedy works for some time; this is also true of a daily remedy.

While certain substances (notably coffee, menthol, camphor, and eucalyptus) can antidote single-dose homeopathic remedies in some sensitive individuals, prescription medications may not interfere with their function. (Topical steroids, antibiotics, and antifungals and oral antibiotics and cortisone products can be suppressive and are best used in consultation with your homeopath.)[230] Be assured, however, that homeopathic remedies do not interfere with the function of conventional medications. Thus, you can pursue homeopathic treatment while continuing your medications or working with your prescribing doctor to phase them out when possible. "Patients with schizophrenia may need to continue their prescription medications along with homeopathic treatment," Dr. Reichenberg-Ullman notes.

As a final note, regarding the efficacy of homeopathy for schizophrenia, she states: "Homeopathic effectiveness is most limited by the skill, knowledge, and experience of the homeopath and the cooperation of the patient. . . . [S]chizophrenia is definitely challenging to treat homeopathically and should only be attempted by a practitioner with considerable experience in both homeopathy and mental health."[231]

As is the case with any medical intervention, results are likely to be better when treatment is initiated early in the course of the illness. One of the difficulties in treating people who have had schizophrenia for years is that the drugs used to keep it under control are very strong and cloud the symptom picture, making it difficult to determine the appropriate homeopathic remedy. "They are so numbing over time," says Dr. Reichenberg-Ullman, that it is very hard to get clear psychological, emotional, and physical symptoms and thus the accurate image of the person needed to identify the constitutional remedy for that individual.

Avoiding substances such as coffee, which can interfere with the action of homeopathic remedies, is recommended, but for patients who are unable to do that, there is a solution. "They are given a daily dose of their remedy," she states.

The results she has seen with schizophrenia and other "mental" illnesses have given Dr. Reichenberg-Ullman a vision for the future. She would like to see homeopathy become standard treatment in both inpatient psychiatric facilities and emergency rooms. In the latter, homeopathy could be used "across the whole spectrum, for everything from trauma to acute psychiatric disturbances," she notes.

 There are more than a thousand classical homeopaths in the United States, a small percentage of whom specialize in mental health. One source to help you find a qualified homeopath in your area is the Homeopathic Academy of Naturopathic Physicians (HANP), 12132 SE Foster Place, Portland, OR 97266; tel: 503-761-3298; website: www.healthy.net/hanp.

Gwen: Homeopathic Zinc

At the age of 56, Gwen had a psychotic break and was put on Stelazine, one of the old class of antipsychotics.* Her troubles began with an increasingly stressful situation at work. An elementary school teacher, she began to be terrified of the principal, a very large woman whom Gwen describes as a "maternal archetype." She felt demeaned by the woman and tried to resolve the situation by keeping her distance, but it seemed that the principal and another teacher were colluding to make Gwen's work life difficult. They interfered with her ability to be effective and to feel satisfaction in her job.

---

* This case study adapted, by permission of Judyth Reichenberg-Ullman, from Judyth Reichenberg-Ullman, N.D., L.C.S.W., and Robert Ullman, N.D., *Prozac Free: Homeopathic Alternatives to Conventional Drug Therapies* (Berkeley, Calif.: North Atlantic Books, 2002), pages 218–21. With update provided through personal communication, 2002.

Her terror increased. "My mouth was completely dry for a whole month," she reports. "I felt adrenaline rushes and found it hard to focus my mind. I couldn't seem to get enough water."

When she was given a class that "didn't want to learn," Gwen was sure that the principal had done this on purpose. Soon, she began to believe that the FBI had bugged her classroom and people were watching her everywhere she went. The latter made it hard for her to be in a public place and she began to avoid it. "I was in utter agony," she recalls. She became convinced that her house was bugged as well, and as a consequence she took to writing notes to her husband instead of talking. Her feelings of being demeaned and diminished increased. It was clear that Gwen had broken under stress and acute psychosis was the result.

After putting her on Stelazine, an antipsychotic, Gwen's psychiatrist urged her to return to Dr. Reichenberg-Ullman, whom she had seen, and been successfully treated by, for a variety of physical complaints over the years. Gwen did so, meanwhile continuing to take the Stelazine, which was helping to reduce her paranoia.

Gwen told Dr. Reichenberg-Ullman that she didn't have good boundaries, that "people's stuff sticks to me." She related a dream she had had in which a solid floor "needed a fire to keep it going. The plywood walls were separating from the solid tongue-and-groove floor." She also reported that her previous complaints of chronic hoarseness, severe headaches, incontinence, and violent belching had returned. In addition, she craved salty food and fruit.

The constitutional remedy indicated for her was *Phosphorus,* which was the remedy she had received before. "This is a medicine for thirsty, sensitive, fearful yet compassionate people who pick up very easily on the thoughts and feelings of those around them," explains Dr. Reichenberg-Ullman.

Gwen was able to discontinue the Stelazine after taking it for a month. A few months later, she had another psychotic episode, although it was milder this time. She again felt terror and anxiety at work, believed that people were thinking about her, and felt the compulsion to try to please people. She stayed home from work for three days and took Stelazine again.

When Dr. Reichenberg-Ullman asked Gwen to identify the overriding psychological issue in her life, she answered: "It's being the victim, the outcast. Separation from my family. I was the black sheep, the scapegoat, the schoolyard victim. I never felt part of the group." She explained that her family moved a lot, which made it hard to develop friends, and within her family, she experienced rejection by her parents, which was the hardest thing of all. Gwen felt great guilt over her inability to please her parents.

Her experiences at the school tapped into these feelings. With the psychotic break, she "had a fear that I was being framed, imprisoned, and condemned for being who I was and for what I was sharing with the children. I felt more and more threatened. I withdrew more and more. I felt shunned, excluded, as if I weren't teaching well."

Schizophrenia can be one of the means by which a person copes with an untenable situation, notes Dr. Reichenberg-Ullman. When a sensitive person encounters a situation such as Gwen did as a child—she could not be accepted for who she was and would have to become someone else to gain acceptance—she must find a way to cope with the irresolvable dilemma. "There is just no way to make sense of what's going on, so she just leaves, and there's a separation of her reality, a whole delusional state that develops," she explains.[232]

After Gwen's second breakdown, Dr. Reichenberg-Ullman gave her the remedy *Zincum metallicum* (zinc), which was indicated by the feeling of being a criminal and a history of restless legs.

Over the next three and a half years, Gwen was fine. On a few occasions, when her paranoia began to return, she repeated doses of the remedy, along with taking Stelazine at a low dose for a short time, and the paranoia subsided.

Later, she told Dr. Reichenberg-Ullman: "I've felt really good, very centered and focused in the classroom, handling a million details. Before, I couldn't keep the thread together. One of my watercolor pieces was even accepted in a show. All the pieces are fitting together. I have my courage, self-respect, and dignity back."

Later still, Gwen was given *Zincum phosphoricum* to address her lingering symptom of incontinence (all her other physical complaints were resolved), since *Phosphorus* had worked so well with that in the past. Over the past five years, Gwen has had to repeat the remedy periodically. On several occasions, when she was under a lot of stress at work, she took a very low dose of Stelazine, but for the past few years none has been needed.

"Her intellect, alertness, and creativity have been excellent, as has her overall degree of happiness and satisfaction," reports Dr. Reichenberg-Ullman. She notes that Gwen never required hospitalization, although without homeopathic treatment, it might have come to that. "Gwen is thoroughly convinced that homeopathy works, and so is her psychiatrist."

Considering the discussion in chapter 4 regarding pyroluric schizophrenia, it is curious that the remedy that worked to dispel Gwen's psychosis was homeopathic zinc, which is the primary nutrient needed in this form of schizophrenia. *Zinc* was prescribed for Gwen, however, based on extensive homeopathic interviews and the emergent constitutional cluster unrelated to the concepts in chapter 4. Once again, a remedy that works well for one person with schizophrenia will not necessarily do the same for another person with schizophrenia. Homeopathic treatment is based entirely on the individual.

Freddie: Stabilizing a Teenager

From the time he was eight years old, Freddie went through periods of wanting to hurt people.*

"I wanted to make them feel scared so they'd know what I was going through," he says. He kept these feelings to himself, knowing that this kind of thinking was odd. At the age of 15, Freddie had a psychotic break, during which he heard voices. He lived in a state of fear—of himself, of other people, and of objects.

---

* This case study adapted, by permission of Judyth Reichenberg-Ullman from Judyth Reichenberg-Ullman, N.D., L.C.S.W., and Robert Ullman, N.D., *Prozac Free: Homeopathic Alternatives to Conventional Drug Therapies* (Berkeley, Calif.: North Atlantic Books, 2002), pages 222–5. With update provided through personal communication.

Afraid that he might hurt himself, he would sit on his hands to keep them from strangling him. He was scared that kids at school would hurt him or cabinets would fall on him or chairs swallow him up. "I see pictures in my head of me getting hurt. My dreams move very fast," he says, adding that until he was put on psychiatric drugs, he didn't know if his dreams were real or not.

Eight months before his breakdown, his mother had observed a disturbing change in him. From a seemingly confident, adventurous boy, he grew "quiet, sullen, gloomy, and secretive." He stayed in his room a lot and wrote on the computer, producing a flood of poetry, mostly about death, some of which was frightening in its depiction of murder. His interests during this time focused on the macabre and the paranormal, from mystery and horror novels to the eerie television show *The X-Files.* To Freddie's mother, it seemed as though her son was in a trance.

He couldn't sleep and became confused and depressed. School was difficult for him because he couldn't concentrate and he didn't want to talk to people. He was preoccupied with thoughts of injury and saw bloody images in his head, including "body parts being thrown into a river."

Alarmed by the way he was acting, school authorities talked to Freddie's mother about getting him help at a children's psychiatric hospital. She did so, and one doctor there prescribed Zoloft and Haldol. A second psychiatrist substituted Risperdal (an atypical antipsychotic, presumed to have fewer side effects than the older class of antipsychotics) for the Haldol. The doctors disagreed on the diagnosis, suggesting schizophrenia, severe depression with psychosis, or bipolar disorder.

On the medication, Freddie's depression eased and his hallucinations stopped. At this point, two months after his psychotic breakdown, his mother took him to Dr. Reichenberg-Ullman. He had stopped taking the drugs a week before, with the support of his psychiatrist. Off the drugs, Freddie was lethargic, weepy, dazed, unable to concentrate, and unable to make it through a day of school. Dr. Reichenberg-Ullman notes that normally she would prefer that a person in Freddie's state continue taking his medications until the appropriate homeopathic remedy could be identified and have a chance to work. This approach makes it more likely that the person will be able to avoid relapse and hospitalization.

"When we saw Freddie for the initial appointment, he reminded us of a terrified deer paralyzed by the headlights at night on a forest road," she recalls. He impressed her as "extremely bright, introspective, creative, and sensitive. We thought it would be a terrible shame for such a brilliant individual to be trapped in a schizophrenic world for life."

Dr. Reichenberg-Ullman prescribed *Thea* (tea), which is indicated for "people who have an unexplainable desire to injure or kill others." This medicine successfully "took the edge off" Freddie's fears for some months. Then, after discovering that he was fascinated with quantum physics and spent a lot of time learning about it, Dr. Reichenberg-Ullman changed his homeopathic remedy to *Hydrogen,* indicated for "extremely deep thinkers and highly sensitive individuals who search intently for the meaning of life. They may soar to blissful states in which they feel integrally connected to the universe, then plunge to the depths of despair and separation." People who need this remedy often exhibit an interest in the stars, planets, black holes, and the "farthest reaches of the universe."

It has now been more than two years since Freddie began homeopathic treatment. He never did need to go back on psychiatric medications nor did he have to be hospitalized. Although he has periods of anxiety and instability, overall he is "relatively stable and able to function," reports Dr. Reichenberg-Ullman. He returned to school, interacted more with others, and was able to get his driver's license and land a summer job. By Freddie's account, he no longer suffered from fear, felt "much more together," and was "doing better in all ways."

Freddie discontinued treatment at this point, although Dr. Reichenberg-Ullman would have preferred regular homeopathic follow-up for at least two more years. However, she adds, "His mother contacted the office a year later to say that Freddie had successfully completed his first year of college and had progressed well in all areas of his life."

8 Conflict and Spirit: Psychosomatic Medicine

While we have seen in this book that biochemical factors play a strong role in schizophrenia, the source of the disturbed biochemistry may not be on the Physical Level. As discussed in chapter 5, such imbalances are often caused by interference on other levels of healing. Here we look at disturbance at the Mental Level of Healing, which in turn can manifest as problems in a person's energetic field or biochemistry or both.

As stated before, to consider the possible role of psychological factors does not signal a return to the former psychological model of bad parenting as the source of schizophrenia. Rather, it acknowledges that body, mind, and spirit are inseparable and that in some individuals, the psychological factors discussed in this chapter may be operational.

Psychosomatic medicine, a European academic discipline, provides a means of understanding interference on the mental plane. In this chapter, Johannes Beckmann, M.D., a general practitioner who specialized in psychosomatic medicine at the University of Toulouse, France, and the University Miguel Cervet in Madrid, describes how an irresolvable conflict in the psyche can result in schizophrenia. In his private practice in Palma de Mallorca, Spain, he integrates this psychological approach to illness with biological medicine (which regards illness as stemming from imbalance in the "internal milieu" or cellular terrain of the body, with treatment operating on the cellular level to restore balance) to attend to the body, mind, and spirit aspects of healing.

As with other medical modalities that focus on addressing the underlying factors in illness, Dr. Beckmann's approach has broad application and he sees patients with a wide range of conditions. While he has treated fewer than 20 people with schizophrenia thus far in his practice, the results of his innovative early work are encouraging. Psychosomatic medicine produced recovery in 20 percent. In the remaining cases, Dr. Beckmann found that over-medication was an impediment to treatment.

This raises two issues of importance to the discussion of natural medicine treatment of schizophrenia. First, the application of many natural medicine techniques to schizophrenia is relatively new. As these techniques begin to be practiced more widely and receive research attention over the next decade, we can expect exciting new advances in the field of treatment.

The second important issue is the damaging effects of medication, as discussed in chapter 1. While antipsychotic drugs may be necessary in some cases, it is sound medical practice to pursue natural treatments that can resolve or ameliorate psychotic symptoms rather than abandon an individual to drugs as the only intervention. Taken for long enough or prescribed irresponsibly, psychiatric drugs may interfere with the efficacy of natural treatments that might otherwise have been beneficial.

What Is Psychosomatic Medicine?

Psychosomatic medicine is an area of specialization in European medical training. While the term also applies to an approach used by some psychiatrists and physicians in the United States, the two forms of psychosomatic medicine are quite different. Among other distinctions, the American approach tends to emphasize behavioral therapies, while European practice focuses on the deeper psychological issues behind illness.

European psychosomatic medicine reflects the simple recognition that the mind and spirit (the Greek *psyche* means "breath, principle of life, soul," and in combination form indicates this along with "mind and mental processes") are integrally connected to and influence the body (*soma* means "body").

A psychosomatic disorder is one in which an internal unresolved conflict finds outlet in the body in what is called a functional disease, according to Dr. Beckmann. Functional disease is distinct from organic disease in that diagnostics such as X rays, blood tests, and electrocardiograms can find none of the measurable changes of organic disease. In functional disease, the functions are being interfered with, but there is no sign of organic disease.

As an example of a psychosomatic disorder, Dr. Beckmann cites a 13-year-old girl who had not yet started to menstruate, but was beginning to look at boys. Her father, noticing this, told her that she should not look at any male aside from him until she was 16. When the girl still did not start menstruating in the next few years, her parents were concerned and took her to the doctor. The doctor determined that everything was fine; she did not have any organic disease that would interfere with menstruation. When she turned 16, released from "the program her father had impressed on her mind and psychic world," she began to menstruate. Freed from the conflict the prohibition posed to her, her body was free to become a woman.

Conflict and the Spirit

In his practice, Dr. Beckmann deals with dilemmas of the mind, body, and spirit. (He notes that "the unconscious and the spirit are the same thing; one word in psychology, another in the religious sciences.") A conflict is at the root of all disorders, according to his model. Often, the conflict relates to childhood experiences. As a child, the person begins to suppress his own wishes, his own self, because when he shows his true self it creates conflict with his father, mother, siblings, or society. The threat of conflict trains the person into an adapted way of life, explains Dr. Beckmann. "The person says, 'I cannot be myself because when I am myself I have problems with others.'"

At first, his spirit finds an outlet in dreams. As the conflict grows stronger, nightmares ensue. This reflects the mounting inner tension of suppressing the spirit, which can also be called the imaginary (imagination is a component of the imaginary). When dreams are remembered, that means the suppression is not complete. Nightmares are the spirit attempting to resolve the

> ## In Their Own Words
>
> *"For me, madness was definitely not a condition of illness; I did not believe that I was ill. It was rather a country, opposed to Reality, where reigned an implacable light. . . ."[233]*
>
> —Renée, a recovered schizophrenic

conflict and remove the blockage. When the nightmares stop and dreams are no longer remembered, this means that the person has adapted to completely suppressing the conflict and to being "a good boy, a good student, the best." The price is suppression of his soul and his feelings.

This pattern was described by psychosomatic medicine clinician and Professor Mahmoud Sami-Ali of the University of Paris as "the pathology of adaptation" or "the pathology of banality." The latter phrase is apt because, without soul or spirit, life is banal, explains Dr. Beckmann. Although this example is a childhood one, the same process occurs whenever the spirit is suppressed in order to "resolve" a conflict. It is not a true resolution, and body, mind, and spirit bear the consequences of the suppression. Internal conflicts that arise in adulthood are related to early childhood conflicts and their attendant messages, according to Dr. Beckmann.

"There is a law in nature that says you attract your similars," he says. "This is a law of physics, where matter attracts matter, and the same happens in the spiritual world," he says. If you have conflict and disorder internally, you attract conflicts that involve similar contradictions. This gives you the opportunity to resolve it this time and "get out of the disorder. We always attract what happens to us."

Dr. Beckmann adds that he believes even babies attract their similars. "They attract this terrible situation or this beautiful situation of family, of parents," he says. "They are not passive. They have an energy, a very powerful energy that attracts also." Viewed from this light, "you understand that the father and the mother are not the culprit or guilty party. This is not to exempt them from responsibility, because they could give the child a better life, but the real origin of the situation is in the person."

The Spirit's Message

In Dr. Beckmann's view, illness, whether schizophrenia or heart disease, arrives when "the development of the spirit has stopped or something that needs to happen is not happening. . . . We are not here to develop a body or psychology; these develop by nature. We are here to develop human consciousness, spirit—it's the same. To develop the behavioral virtues connected to this— to behave with wisdom, kindness, compassion, all the things that are related to love or justice, to purity, to connection with spirit."

Schizophrenia and other disorders, then, can be seen as the spirit's attempt to tell you something. Each form of response has its logic. Dr. Beckmann explains that the nature of the conflict dictates the manifestation. For example, physical symptoms relate to the stage of development during which the conflict originated. "Every organ or system in the body has its moment in the time loop. You would look at when the affected

In Dr. Beckmann's view, illness, whether schizophrenia or heart disease, arrives when "the development of the spirit has stopped or something that needs to happen is not happening. . . . We are not here to develop a body or psychology; these develop by nature. We are here to develop human consciousness, spirit—it's the same." Schizophrenia and other disorders, then, can be seen as the spirit's attempt to tell you something.

organ or system develops in the life of a child, then you would know when the conflict started."

In psychosomatic disorders, "the mind can't face the conflict and the imaginary helps to solve the conflict through the body in the form of functional disease." When the conflict is too great and the suppression is complete and goes on for too long, organic disease results. "Organic disease is the last development of the pathology of banality, of adaptation," says Dr. Beckmann.

In terms of "mental" disorders, the manifestation relates to the options contained in the conflict. In depression, the person waits for the solution to the internal conflict to come from outside, "doing nothing, staying there, waiting." In neuroses, such as obsessive-compulsive or anxiety disorders, the nature of the dilemma is that a solution exists, there are at least two choices and one of them offers a way out of the internal conflict, but the person doesn't act on it.

"This is the definition of neurotic," states Dr. Beckmann. "It is the conflict with the possibility of a solution, but the person stays in the continuous dilemma." An example is wanting to separate from a partner that you know for your mental, physical, and spiritual well-being you need to leave, and you have the financial and circumstantial wherewithal to do it, but you don't.

In the case of one woman in this position, for years she thought to herself every day, "Soon I'll go." Then her husband had a stroke and half of his body was paralyzed. She could no longer play with the possibility of going, and now told herself, "I must stay. I now have no choice." The internal conflict was still there, however. With the continued suppression of her spirit, organic disease developed. Six months later, she had developed a brain tumor.

Another of Dr. Beckmann's patients experienced a trauma that, if her spirit had been suppressed, would have led to depression, anxiety attacks, or even organic disease. Instead, something different happened. This woman found out, after 20 years of marriage, that her husband had been cheating on her the whole time and had had lots of other women. She had thought all those years that she was the only one. "She was in shock after she found out," says Dr. Beckmann, "but she did not get ill because, although she loved her husband, she existed independently of him and had a strong relationship to a higher power. She did not get ill because her husband was not her life's source and as a result she did not experience the situation as an extreme conflict." Her spirit was not suppressed, so she could find her way out of a potential dilemma by not defining it as a dilemma at all.

"When organic disease occurs, there is always an old conflict that brought the person in the past into the pathology of suppression and adaptation. The spirit is, in this case, asleep," which is the means of managing the conflict, explains Dr. Beckmann. "When a new, extreme conflict arises, organic disease is the next step in managing it. The adapted person has no other resources for handling the conflict." By contrast, in neuroses and psychoses, the spirit or the imaginary is less suppressed and the inner conflict finds an outlet through the mind.

In the case of schizophrenia, taking leave of one's mind is perceived as the only means of escape from the conflict, an eventuality mentioned by Dr. Reichenberg-Ullman in the previous chapter. Dr. Beckmann tells of a Russian woman who was brought to Spain by a man upon whom she was completely dependent (her pattern was dependence). He came home drunk every night and beat her. She could not go back to Russia and she could not stay where she was. "This was a conflict that could only be solved through her mind. The only way to solve it was to go crazy," Dr. Beckman explains. In psychosis, the imaginary has not been completely suppressed and is strong enough to provide an outlet through the mind. "The psyche finds the solution in the nonreality," says Dr. Beckmann.

In neurosis, the ongoing conflict from which the person fails to extricate herself interferes with the individual living to her full potential, to the fullest life of her spirit. In psychosis, the disorder in the psyche has the same effect. Dr. Beckmann notes that the antipsychotic drugs used to "treat" schizophrenia and other psychoses suppress the imaginary, which further restricts the spirit and opens the way to the development of organic disease, compounding the already significant problem of schizophrenia.

On the physical level, the effects of psychosis go beyond disturbed biochemistry, says Dr. Beckmann, citing the work of his mentor, German researcher and physician Ryke Geerd Hamer, M.D., who studied the link between traumatic events (which include the onset of an inner conflict) and the development of illness. The contradiction or conflict actually creates blockages in the brain, with different kinds of conflict affecting different areas in the brain.

Normally, if there is a problem in one hemisphere of the brain, the other hemisphere can compensate. With schizophrenia, however, there is blockage in both hemispheres and in different places. The sites of blockage determine the kind of schizophrenia that manifests. For example, catatonic schizophrenia has blockages in different locations from those of paranoid schizophrenia.

 Resources

Dr. Hamer's work is widely known in Europe. If you read German, an Internet search on his name will give you many choices for learning more about his pioneering approach to medicine. Some English translations are available; contact Quintessenz, Box 39510, 374 Lakeshore Road East, Mississauga, Ontario, L5G 4S6 Canada; tel/fax: 905-271-8047.

Psychosomatic Treatment

Unlike psychoanalysis, psychosomatic medicine often produces fast results. By homing in on the internal conflict behind the illness, the issue can often be resolved in one or two sessions. While there may be childhood conflicts that relate to the most recent catalyzing conflict, it is not necessary to uncover all of those in order to release the mind from the schizophrenia crisis. The tendency to become ill in this way remains, however, says Dr. Beckmann. "The patient just learns to handle the basic conflict and avoid schizophrenic life situations."

After recognizing the conflict, it may take the person some time to act on a solution, but identifying it can do a lot to ease the mind. Some people choose to continue psychosomatic analysis in order to explore deeper psychological and spiritual issues, but the initial problem can often find quick resolution.

In the case of schizophrenia, it might take longer to remove or resolve one side of the conflictual equation in order to provide the mind with an escape route aside from madness. In some instances, however, the solution is relatively simple, as occurred with Madeleine, once the truth was uncovered.

Madeleine: Resolving a Psychic Dilemma

Madeleine, 32, was diagnosed with schizophrenia a year and a half before she came to Dr. Beckmann. Her breakdown was severe enough to require a stay in a psychiatric hospital, where she was put on heavy antipsychotics. After she was discharged, she was under the care of a psychiatrist. For the next year, she took the drugs he prescribed, but she was so disturbed by how they made her feel that she finally stopped taking them.

Not long after, her husband observed that her symptoms were starting up again, that she was imagining things and losing touch with reality. She didn't think she was in as bad a shape as he thought she was, but he was afraid she was headed for another breakdown and wanted her to get help. As Madeleine didn't want to go back on the medication, she went to Dr. Beckmann.

To begin the search for the conflict, he asked Madeleine what was going on in her life in the period just before her breakdown. Madeleine talked of a problem she had been having at the little butcher shop she ran. She rented the space and her landlord and his family lived above the store. She began to notice signs of someone having been in her shop after hours. When she would come in at the start of her work day, things would not be exactly where she had left them and it would be clear that someone had gone through her papers. It happened numerous times and she suspected that someone in the landlord's family was looking for money. As she never left money there, she lost nothing, but she didn't like someone being in her shop when she wasn't there. (You might say that this is typical of the onset of paranoia, but the resolution of her illness showed that her illness actually started later.)

She was afraid to talk to the landlord and didn't want to bother her husband with this problem. She ran the shop by herself, and he had his own work to contend with. So this was a conflict from which she saw no escape. Her schizophrenia provided an escape, however, in that she could not work and had to close her business. But ending the conflict had not resolved her illness.

"I knew there was another problem," Dr. Beckmann said, but Madeleine couldn't recall any other conflict in her life at the time. After he asked her to think again about what had happened before her first breakdown, she suddenly remembered something else. "Oh, yes, I went to a psychic," she said. At that, she began to cry.

She had consulted a psychic in the hopes of getting some guidance as to what to do about the situation. She had consulted psychics before and had great faith in them. She told the psychic, "I've come because of my work. If you see anything bad about my life, please don't tell me."

The psychic irresponsibly disregarded this request. The first thing she said was, "I see your husband dead," and she added that it would happen soon. Madeleine was shocked by this revelation. Her husband, who was an aggressive man, was her protector. He was the one who would return her sense of security at the store if she asked him to deal with her problem. She hadn't called upon him to do so, but she always knew that he was there and would protect her. She depended on him.

As she firmly believed in psychics, she did not question the prediction. "When she heard that he was going to die, it was at that exact moment that the schizophrenic conflict began," says Dr. Beckmann. There was no escaping his death, and she felt she couldn't live without him. The problems at the shop were secondary to losing her husband. From that moment on, she began to have auditory hallucinations, which escalated to the point of complete delirium, and she had to be hospitalized.

After Madeleine told Dr. Beckmann about the psychic, he pointed out that it had been a year and a half since the prediction and her husband was not dead. He asked if her husband was ill. Madeleine replied that he was not, but that she lived in fear of him having a fatal accident. "You could see her fear," recalls Dr. Beckmann, "and all of this because a psychic said her husband would die soon."

Dr. Beckmann tried the tactic then of talking about what a psychic is and how clairvoyants have existed throughout history, but that didn't signify that they are all-wise and all-knowing. "I was explaining this to the woman when a look of amazement appeared on her face, and she said, 'There is something I'm not telling you.'"

She had suddenly remembered that a month after her session with the psychic, she had gone with her husband and a friend who worked for a film crew to a set for a Western they were filming. They had put her husband in the movie as a cowboy extra. In the scene, her husband was in the town saloon when another cowboy came in and shot him dead.

The conflict was resolved. Her husband was indeed "dead," as the psychic had predicted. Madeleine no longer had to live in fear. "From that moment on, she had no schizophrenia," says Dr. Beckmann. The symptoms that had begun again when she went off the drugs disappeared and there was no need to go back on medication. Now, five years later, Madeleine is secretary and receptionist for a small company and is still free of psychiatric symptoms and medication.

In the interim, she worked on her belief that she can't live without her husband protector. The existence of that belief indicated that spirit was excluded in her life, despite her belief in psychic readers, Dr. Beckmann explains. "Without spirit, without independence and consciousness of the self, you cannot heal fully. We must make the connection between body, mind, and spirit. If you don't bring in the spirit, you don't have healing."

9 The Shamanic View of Mental Illness

As discussed in chapter 5, interferences that manifest as schizophrenia can occur on any of the Five Levels of Healing. Earlier chapters focused on the physical and electromagnetic levels and the application of biochemical and energy medicine, among other modalities. In the previous chapter, Dr. Beckmann's work in psychosomatic medicine centered on interferences at the mental level and the importance of the spirit in psychological well-being.

This chapter addresses disturbances that arise on the fourth level of healing, the Intuitive Level. This is the psychic dimension, where forces outside of oneself can affect one's well-being. Shamanic or psychic healing is the intervention that operates at this level to remove or reconcile the foreign energies that are creating disturbance and manifesting as schizophrenia.

By addressing the foreign energy, shamanic healing helps to bring body, mind, and spirit back into alignment. As with other energy-based medicine, the goal is the same: the clearing of negative influences and blockages, and the restoration of balance, wholeness, and connectedness.

In addition to its useful analysis of energetic issues, shamanic tradition offers a view of mental disorders that is sorely lacking in the Western world and that holds the key to a whole other way of healing. Disregard of this view has led to treatment based on suppression of symptoms, rather than therapeutic methods that bring

What Is Shamanic Healing?

Shamanism is "perhaps the oldest form of practical spirituality in the world, originating in the time of Ice Age people, going back as far as 35,000 B.C."[234] It is also practiced virtually everywhere in the world. A shaman is someone who has gone through advanced initiation into the "hidden" realm. The shaman uses the knowledge gained from the other realm for healing and the good of the community. Shamanic healing is psychic healing, but the term delineates, in particular, indigenous healing that is rooted in traditional ritual.

the body, mind, and spirit back together. In the shamanic view, mental illness signals "the birth of a healer," explains Malidoma Patrice Somé, Ph.D., an internationally celebrated African shaman, diviner, and teacher. Thus, mental disorders are spiritual emergencies, spiritual crises, and need to be regarded as such to aid the healer in being born.

Shamanic traditions around the globe subscribe to this view and the West could benefit greatly from absorbing its wisdom. As psychologist and anthropologist Holger Kalweit writes, "If we were able to understand sickness and suffering as processes of physical and psychic transformation, as do Asian peoples and tribal cultures, we would gain a deeper and less biased view of psychosomatic and psychospiritual processes and begin to realize the many opportunities presented by suffering. . . ."[235]

What a Shaman Sees in a Mental Hospital

Dr. Somé is a member of the Dagara tribe, which is from an area situated at the intersection of Ghana, the Ivory Coast, and Burkina Faso (formerly Upper Volta) in western Africa. Dr. Somé left his homeland to study in Europe and the United States and holds three master's degrees and two doctorates from the Sorbonne and Brandeis University. He has authored two books, *Ritual: Power, Healing, and Community* and *Of Water and the Spirit.*

The latter is his moving autobiography, which tells of his kidnap at the age of four by Jesuit missionaries who kept him prisoner and trained him as a missionary until at 20 he managed to escape. After an arduous trip back to his village, he underwent an initiation that restored him to his people and opened the way to his shamanic practice. Now dedicated to bringing the healing wisdom of the Dagara tribe to the West, he conducts workshops and classes around the world, while still maintaining a close connection with his village in Burkina Faso.

What those in the West view as mental illness, the Dagara people regard as "good news from the other world." The person going through the crisis has been chosen as a medium for a message to the community that needs to be communicated from the spirit realm. "Mental disorder, behavioral disorder of all kinds, signal the fact that two obviously incompatible energies have merged into the same field," says Dr. Somé. These disturbances result when the person does not get assistance in dealing with the presence of the energy from the spirit realm.

One of the things Dr. Somé encountered when he first came to the United States in 1980 for graduate study was how this country deals with mental illness. When a fellow student was sent to a mental institute due to "nervous depression," Dr. Somé went to visit him.

"I was so shocked. That was the first time I was brought face to face with what is done here to people exhibiting the same symptoms I've seen in my village." What struck Dr. Somé was that the attention given to such symptoms was based on pathology, on the idea that the condition is something that needs to stop. This was in complete opposition to the way his culture views such a situation. As he looked around the stark ward at the patients, some in straitjackets, some zoned out on medications, others screaming, he observed to himself, "So this is how the healers who are attempting to be born are treated in this culture. What a loss! What a loss that a person who is finally being aligned with a power from the other world is just being wasted."

Another way to say this, which may make more sense to the Western mind, is that we in the West are not trained in how to deal with or even taught to acknowledge the existence of psychic phenomena, the spiritual world. In fact, psychic abilities are denigrated. When energies from the spiritual world emerge in a Western psyche, that individual is completely unequipped to integrate them or even recognize what is happening. The result can be terrifying. Without the proper context for and assistance in dealing with the breakthrough from another level of reality, for all practical purposes, the person is insane. Heavy dosing with antipsychotic drugs compounds the problem and prevents the integration that could lead to soul development and growth in the individual who has received these energies.

> **We in the West are not trained in how to deal with or even taught to acknowledge the existence of psychic phenomena, the spiritual world. When energies from the spiritual world emerge in a Western psyche, that individual is completely unequipped to integrate them or even recognize what is happening. The result can be terrifying. Without the proper context for and assistance in dealing with the breakthrough from another level of reality, for all practical purposes, the person is insane.**

On the mental ward, Dr. Somé saw a lot of "beings" hanging around the patients, "entities" that are invisible to most people but that shamans and some psychics are able to see. "They were causing the crisis in these people," he says. It appeared to him that these beings were trying to get the medications and their effects out of the bodies of the people the beings were trying to merge with, and were increasing the patients' pain in the process. "The beings were acting almost like some kind of excavator in the energy field of the people. They were really fierce about that. The people they were doing that to were just screaming and yelling," he said. He couldn't stay in that environment and had to leave.

In the Dagara tradition, the community helps the person reconcile the energies of both worlds—"the world of the spirit that he or she is merged with, and the village and community." That person is able then to serve as a bridge between the worlds and help the living with information and healing they need. Thus, the spiritual crisis ends with the birth of another healer. "The other world's relationship with our world is one of sponsorship," Dr. Somé explains. "More often than not, the knowledge and skills that arise from this kind of merger are a knowledge or a skill that is provided directly from the other world."

> ## In Their Own Words
>
> "My illness is a journey of fear. . . . Sometimes I feel I can't stand it any longer. It hurts too much. . . . It seems, at these times, when I reach bottom, that I'm given a message and I feel mystical, spiritual, and like a prophet who must tell anyone that there's really nothing to fear. . . . I somehow feel better for being the courier."[236]
>
> —An artist, 37, diagnosed with paranoid schizophrenia

The beings who were increasing the pain of the inmates on the mental hospital ward were actually attempting to merge with the inmates in order to get messages through to this world. The people they had chosen to merge with were getting no assistance in learning how to be a bridge between the worlds and the beings' attempts to merge were thwarted. The result was the sustaining of the initial disorder of energy and the aborting of the birth of a healer.

"The Western culture has consistently ignored the birth of the healer," states Dr. Somé. "Consequently, there will be a tendency from the other world to keep trying as many people as possible in an attempt to get somebody's attention. They have to try harder." The spirits are drawn to people whose senses have not been anesthetized. "The sensitivity is pretty much read as an invitation to come in," he notes.

Those who develop so-called mental disorders are those who are sensitive, which is viewed in Western culture as oversensitivity.

Indigenous cultures don't see it that way and, as a result, sensitive people don't experience themselves as overly sensitive. In the West, "it is the overload of the culture they're in that is just wrecking them," observes Dr. Somé. The frenetic pace, the bombardment of the senses, and the violent energy that characterize Western culture can overwhelm sensitive people.

The Science of the Energy Field

The foreign energy addressed in shamanic healing enters the energy field that surrounds the body, which is also called the aura. While, unlike shamans, laypeople cannot typically see their aura, they receive evidence of its existence all the time. Have you ever "felt your skin crawl" when you met someone new? Have you ever suddenly and for no apparent reason felt drained or depressed when you walked into a room of people? These reactions are the result of discordant foreign energies entering your energy field, or aura, where they are not a good match with your energy and consequently produce a sense of unease or discomfort. These foreign energies can be beings from the spirit realm or energies in your environment.

Energy influences may not be transitory. The energy field around your body is subtle and fragile and can actually be damaged, which renders it more permeable to foreign energies and more likely that they will remain. Among the events or practices that can damage or pollute the aura are emotional or physical trauma, psychic or verbal abuse, other people's negative or bad thoughts about you, and substance abuse. To help in understanding energy and the aura, think of the aura as an opaque cloud that surrounds the body and the foreign energies as dust and dirt that collect in the cloud. The more foreign energies the person is exposed to, the more dusty and dirty the cloud becomes, the more clogged the energy field or aura. With too much buildup of dust and dirt, energy flow is compromised and the person's health begins to suffer.

Physicians and psychics alike have noted that the energy field can be occupied by energies that produce mental, emotional, and physical symptoms and, if allowed to remain, can lead to disease.[237] Psychiatrist Shakuntala Modi, M.D., of Wheeling, West Virginia, has been researching energy field disturbances for more than 15 years. She has identified a range of physical and psychological symptoms and conditions that result from such disturbances, including schizophrenia, panic disorders, depression, headaches, allergies, uterine disorders, weight gain, and stammering. Further, under clinical hypnotherapy, 77 out of 100 patients cited foreign "beings" in their aura as responsible for the symptoms or condition for which they were pursuing treatment.

Dr. Modi's research revealed that these beings are "the most common cause of depression" and "the single leading cause of psychiatric problems in general."[238] Dr. Modi also found that after removing the foreign energies from the patient's energy field using hypnotherapy, the patient's symptoms "often cleared up immediately."[239]

The concept of energy disturbances in a person's energy field causing a variety of physical and psychological problems is gaining greater recognition and acceptance in the healing professions and among the public at large. A simple way to look at the issue of "energy pollution" is that, like the environment and your body, your energy field is subject to toxic buildup (the dust and dirt analogy) and requires cleansing to restore it to health. Just as we take measures to clean up our planet and engage in various body detoxification methods such as fasts or colonics, we need to take steps to clear the toxins from our auras.

Shamanic healing is a method for cleansing your energy field of the toxins that are interfering with your physical, emotional, and spiritual health. Or in the case of a spirit being trying to merge with you for healing purposes, shamanic practice brings your energy and that of the spirit being into alignment, thus resolving the symptoms resulting from discordant energy and realizing the potential for individual growth.

Schizophrenia and Foreign Energy

With schizophrenia, there is a special "receptivity to a flow of images and information, which cannot be controlled," states Dr.

Somé. "When this kind of rush occurs at a time that is not personally chosen, and particularly when it comes with images that are scary and contradictory, the person goes into a frenzy."

What is required in this situation is first to separate the person's energy from the extraneous foreign energies, by using shamanic practice (what is known as a "sweep") to clear the latter out of the individual's aura. With the clearing of their energy field, the person no longer picks up a flood of information and so no longer has a reason to be scared and disturbed, explains Dr. Somé.

Then it is possible to help the person align with the energy of the spirit being attempting to come through from the other world and give birth to the healer. The blockage of that emergence is what creates problems. "The energy of the healer is a high-voltage energy," he observes. "When it is blocked, it just burns up the person. It's like a short-circuit. Fuses are blowing. This is why it can be really scary, and I understand why this culture prefers to confine these people. Here they are yelling and screaming, and they're put into a straitjacket. That's a sad image." Again, the shamanic approach is to work on aligning the energies so there is no blockage, "fuses" aren't blowing, and the person can become the healer they are meant to be.

It needs to be noted at this point, however, that not all of the spirit beings that enter a person's energetic field are there for the purposes of promoting healing. There are negative energies as well, which are undesirable presences in the aura. In those cases, the shamanic approach is to remove them from the aura, rather than work to align the discordant energies.

Alex: Crazy in the USA, Healer in Africa

To test his belief that the shamanic view of mental illness holds true in the Western world as well as in indigenous cultures, Dr. Somé took a mental patient back to Africa with him, to his village. "I was prompted by my own curiosity to find out whether there's truth in the universality that mental illness could be connected with an alignment with a being from another world," says Dr. Somé.

Alex was an 18-year-old American who had suffered a psychotic break when he was 14. He had hallucinations, was suicidal, and went through cycles of dangerously severe depression. He was in a mental hospital and had been given a lot of drugs, but nothing was helping. "The parents had done everything—unsuccessfully," says Dr. Somé. "They didn't know what else to do."

With their permission, Dr. Somé took their son to Africa. "After eight months there, Alex had become quite normal, Dr. Somé reports. He was even able to participate with healers in the business of healing; sitting with them all day long and helping them, assisting them in what they were doing with their clients. . . . He spent about four years in my village." Alex stayed by choice, not because he needed more healing. He felt "much safer in the village than in America."

To bring his energy and that of the being from the spiritual realm into alignment, Alex went through a shamanic ritual designed for that purpose, although it was slightly different from the one used with the Dagara people. "He wasn't born in the village, so something else applied. But the result was similar, even though the ritual was not literally the same," explains Dr. Somé. The fact that aligning the energy worked to heal Alex demonstrated to Dr. Somé that the connection between other beings and mental illness is indeed universal.

After the ritual, Alex began to share the messages that the spirit being had for this world. Unfortunately, the people he was talking to didn't speak English (Dr. Somé was away at that point). The whole experience led, however, to Alex's going to college to study psychology. He returned to the United States after four years because "he discovered that all the things that he needed to do had been done, and he could then move on with his life."

The last that Dr. Somé heard was that Alex was in graduate school in psychology at Harvard. No one had thought he would ever be able to complete undergraduate studies, much less get an advanced degree.

Dr. Somé sums up what Alex's mental illness was all about: "He was reaching out. It was an emergency call. His job and his purpose was to be a healer. He said no one was paying attention to that."

After seeing how well the shamanic approach worked for Alex, Dr. Somé concluded that spirit beings are just as much an issue in the West as in his community in Africa. "Yet the question still remains, the answer to this problem must be found here, instead of having to go all the way overseas to seek the answer. There has to be a way in which a little bit of attention beyond the pathology of this whole experience leads to the possibility of coming up with the proper ritual to help people."

Longing for Spiritual Connection

A common thread that Dr. Somé has noticed in "mental" disorders in the West is "a very ancient ancestral energy that has been placed in stasis, that finally is coming out in the person." His job then is to trace it back, to go back in time to discover what that spirit is. In most cases, the spirit is connected to nature, especially with mountains or big rivers, he says.

In the case of mountains, as an example to explain the phenomenon, "it's a spirit of the mountain that is walking side by side with the person and, as a result, creating a time-space distortion that is affecting the person caught in it." What is needed is a merger or alignment of the two energies, "so the person and the mountain spirit become one." Again, the shaman conducts a specific ritual to bring about this alignment.

Dr. Somé believes that he encounters this situation so often in the United States because "most of the fabric of this country is made up of the energy of the machine, and the result of that is the disconnection and the severing of the past. You can run from the past, but you can't hide from it." The ancestral spirit of the natural world comes visiting. "It's not so much what the spirit wants as it is what the person wants," he says. "The spirit sees in us a call for something grand, something that will make life meaningful, and so the spirit is responding to that."

That call, which we don't even know we are making, reflects "a strong longing for a profound connection, a connection that transcends materialism and possession of things and moves into a tangible cosmic dimension. Most of this longing is unconscious, but for spirits, conscious or unconscious doesn't make any difference." They respond to either.

As part of the ritual to merge the mountain and human energy, those who are receiving the "mountain energy" are sent to a mountain area of their choice, where they pick up a stone that calls to them. They bring that stone back for the rest of the ritual and then keep it as a companion; some even carry it around with them. "The presence of the stone does a lot in tuning the perceptive ability of the person," notes Dr. Somé. "They receive all kinds of information that they can make use of, so it's like they get some tangible guidance from the other world as to how to live their life."

When it is the "river energy," those being called go to the river and, after speaking to the river spirit, find a water stone to bring back for the same kind of ritual as with the mountain spirit.

"People think something extraordinary must be done in an extraordinary situation like this," he says. That's not usually the case. Sometimes it is as simple as carrying a stone.

A Sacred Ritual Approach to Mental Illness

One of the gifts a shaman can bring to the Western world is to help people rediscover ritual, which is so sadly lacking. "The abandonment of ritual can be devastating. From the spiritual viewpoint, ritual is inevitable and necessary if one is to live," Dr. Somé writes in *Ritual: Power, Healing, and Community.* "To say that ritual is needed in the industrialized world is an understatement. We have seen in my own people that it is probably impossible to live a sane life without it."[240]

Dr. Somé did not feel that the rituals from his traditional village could simply be transferred to the West, so over his years of shamanic work here, he has designed rituals that meet the very different needs of this culture. Although the rituals change according to the individual or the group involved, he finds that there is a need for certain rituals in general.

One of these involves helping people discover that their distress is coming from the fact that they are "called by beings from the other world to cooperate with them in doing healing work." Ritual allows them to move out of the distress and accept that calling.

Another ritual need relates to initiation. In indigenous cultures all over the world, young people are initiated into adulthood when they reach a certain age. The lack of such initiation in the West is part of the crisis that people are in here, says Dr. Somé. He urges communities to bring together "the creative juices of people who have had this kind of experience, in an attempt to come up with some kind of an alternative ritual that would at least begin to put a dent in this kind of crisis."

Another ritual that repeatedly speaks to the needs of those coming to him for help entails making a bonfire, and then putting into the bonfire "items that are symbolic of issues carried inside the individuals. . . . It might be the issues of anger and frustration against an ancestor who has left a legacy of murder and enslavement or anything, things that the descendant has to live with," he explains. "If these are approached as things that are blocking the human imagination, the person's life purpose, and even the person's view of life as something that can improve, then it makes sense to begin thinking in terms of how to turn that blockage into a roadway that can lead to something more creative and more fulfilling."

The example of issues with an ancestor touches on rituals designed by Dr. Somé that address a serious dysfunction in Western society and in the process "trigger enlightenment" in participants. These are ancestral rituals, and the dysfunction they are aimed at is the mass turning-of-the-back on ancestors. Some of the spirits trying to come through, as described earlier, may be "ancestors who want to merge with a descendant in an attempt to heal what they weren't able to do while in their physical body."

"Unless the relationship between the living and the dead is in balance, chaos ensues," he says. "The Dagara believe that, if such an imbalance exists, it is the duty of the living to heal their ancestors. If these ancestors are not healed, their sick energy will haunt the souls and psyches of those who are responsible for helping them."[241] The rituals focus on healing the relationship with our ancestors, both specific issues of an individual ancestor and the larger cultural issues contained in our past. Dr. Somé has seen extraordinary healing occur at these rituals.

Taking a sacred ritual approach to mental illness rather than regarding the person as a pathological case gives the person affected—and indeed the community at large—the opportunity to begin looking at it from that vantage point too, which leads to "a whole plethora of opportunities and ritual initiative that can be very, very beneficial to everyone present," states Dr. Somé.

Afterword

The Natural Medicine Guide to Schizophrenia places the syndrome known as schizophrenia (which, remember, is not a distinct disease) in the context in which it properly belongs: as a condition that has no single cause but can be brought about by a wide array of factors, from biochemical imbalances to allergies to energy disturbances to psychospiritual interferences, often acting in combination. To approach the treatment of schizophrenia from this context makes recovery a possibility, rather than an improbability.

Understanding illness in the natural medicine model means putting together all the pieces—physical, emotional, psychological, and spiritual—that are contributing to the illness in a particular person. Inherent to the natural medicine approach is the knowledge that body, mind, and spirit are wholly interrelated, such that an imbalance or interference in one affects the others and can produce symptoms in all three areas. For treatment to be effective, it must treat the whole person.

Approaching the treatment of schizophrenia as a matter of putting together the pieces, identifying all of the underlying imbalances and systematically addressing them, can help dispel some of the pain, confusion, fear, and despair raised by receiving such a serious diagnosis as schizophrenia. With steps to take to reduce the environmental stressors—the body, mind, and spirit factors—that contribute to the disorder, people with schizophrenia and their families have active options, in contrast to the passive acceptance of the widely touted view that drugs are the only course available. This book makes it clear that there are many other courses to take and much more positive prognoses.

Treating the whole person and working to restore health on all levels offers the possibility of ameliorating or even reversing the symptoms of schizophrenia. The goal of this approach is not maintenance, but restoring health in body, mind, and spirit and in so doing returning the individual to full participation in life.

Natural medicine therapies offer a future in which the monikers of fear—the "S" word and "cancer of the mind"—lose their relevance and become relics of the past as schizophrenia becomes known as a treatable condition.

May the information in this book enable those with schizophrenia to leave the debilitating aspects of their illness behind and live to their greatest potential.

Appendix A
Professional Degrees and Titles

D.C.	Doctor of Chiropractic
D.D.S.	Doctor of Dental Science/Surgery
D.M.D.	Doctor of Dental Medicine
D.O.	Doctor of Osteopathy
L.Ac.	Licensed Acupuncturist
L.C.S.W.	Licensed Clinical Social Worker
N.D.	Doctor of Naturopathy

Appendix B
Resources

Practitioners in This Book

Johannes Beckmann, M.D.
E-mail: johanbe@terra.es

Dr. Beckmann is a general practitioner and master of psychosomatic medicine (a European degree and medical specialty). His private practice in Palma de Mallorca, Spain, integrates biological medicine, a psychological approach to illness, and body-work therapy.

Lina Garcia, D.D.S., D.M.D.
1443 West Schaumburg Road
Schaumburg, IL 60194
Tel: (847) 985-1777 x39
E-mail: linagarciaj@hotmail.com

Dr. Garcia practices holistic dentistry and holistic healing with a primary modality of cranial osteopathic diagnosis and treatment.

Dietrich Klinghardt, M.D., Ph.D.
1200 112th Avenue NE, Suite A100
Bellevue, WA 98004
Tel: (425) 688-8818

Dr. Klinghardt specializes in Neural Therapy, Applied Psychoneurobiology, and Family Systems Therapy to address energy disturbances and the transgenerational energy legacies at the root of illness.

Michael Lesser, M.D.
2340 Parker Street
Berkeley, CA 94704
Tel: (510) 845-0700
Website: www.nutritionvitamintherapy.com

A doctor of orthomolecular medicine, Dr. Lesser has 40 years of experience in treating schizophrenia and other disorders with the orthomolecular approach. He is the author of *Nutrition and Vitamin Therapy* and *The Brain Chemistry Diet.*

Devi S. Nambudripad, M.D., D.C., L.Ac., Ph.D.
Pain Clinic
6714 Beach Boulevard
Nambudripad Allergy Research Foundation
6732 Beach Boulevard
Buena Park, CA 90621
Tel: (714) 523-8900
Website: www.naet.com

The Pain Clinic treats various allergy and pain disorders using NAET (Nambudripad's Allergy Elimination Techniques), acupuncture, and chiropractic. The Allergy Research Foundation is a nonprofit organization devoted to conducting clinical trials and studies on NAET and educating the public and professionals alike. Dr. Nambudripad is the author of numerous books, including *Say Goodbye to Illness.*

Judyth Reichenberg-Ullman, N.D., L.C.S.W.
The Northwest Center for Homeopathic Medicine
131 Third Avenue North
Edmonds, WA 98020
Tel: (425) 774-5599
Website: www.healthyhomeopathy.com

In practice with her husband, Robert Ullman, Dr. Reichenberg-Ullman is a licensed naturopathic physician board certified in homeopathy. She has been practicing for 18 years and is the author/coauthor of six books on homeopathic medicine, including *Prozac Free, Ritalin-Free Kids,* and *Whole Woman Homeopathy.*

Hugh D. Riordan, M.D.

Center for the Improvement of Human Functioning International
3100 North Hillside
Wichita, KS 67219
Tel: (316) 682-3100
Website: www.brightspot.org

Dr. Riordan, author of *Medical Mavericks, Volumes I and II,* has practiced "individualized medicine" for over 40 years. He is president of the Center for the Improvement of Human Functioning International, a nonprofit medical, research, and educational organization, which includes the Olive Garvey Center for Healing Arts. Evaluation and treatment focuses on discovering and correcting the underlying biochemical causes of illness.

Malidoma Patrice Somé, Ph.D.

236 West East Avenue, Suite A, PMB 199
Chico, CA 95926
Tel: (530) 894-0740
E-mail: rowenap@jps.net (Rowena Pantaleon, Dr. Somé's assistant)
Website: www.malidoma.com and www.villagewisdom.net

Dr. Somé is an African shaman, diviner, and teacher who brings the healing wisdom of the Dagara tribe to the West.

William J. Walsh, Ph.D.

Health Research Institute and Pfeiffer Treatment Center
4575 Weaver Parkway
Warrenville, IL 60555
Tel: (630) 505-0300
E-mail: info@hriptc.org
Website: www.hriptc.org

Dr. Walsh is the chief scientist/biochemical researcher at HRI-PTC, a nonprofit organization based in Illinois, with services in Minnesota, Maryland, Arizona, and California. A collaboration between medical doctors, biochemists, and nutritionists, the outpatient clinic offers individualized nutrient therapy for schizophrenia, bipolar disorder, autism, ADD, depression, and other conditions.

Organizations

Canadian Schizophrenia Foundation
International Society of Orthomolecular Medicine
16 Florence Avenue
Toronto, Ontario M2N 1E9
Canada
Tel: (416) 733-2117
Website: www.orthomed.org

National Alliance for the Mentally Ill (NAMI)
Colonial Place Three
2101 Wilson Blvd., Suite 300
Arlington, VA 22201
Tel: (800) 950-NAMI
Website: www.nami.org

National Alliance for Research on Schizophrenia and Depression (NARSAD)
60 Cutter Mill Road
Great Neck, NY 11021
Tel: (800) 829-8289 or (516) 829-0091
Website: www.mhsource.com/narsad.html

World Fellowship for Schizophrenia and Allied Disorders
124 Merton Street, Suite 507
Toronto, Ontario M4W 2H2
Canada
Tel: (416) 961-2855
Website: www.world-schizophrenia.org

Endnotes

Introduction

1. C. J. L. Murray, and A. D. Lopez, eds., *Summary: The Global Burden of Disease: A Comprehensive Assessment of Mortality and Disability from Diseases, Injuries, and Risk Factors in 1990 and Projected to 2020* (Cambridge: Harvard School of Public Health on Behalf of the World Health Organization and the World Bank, Harvard University Press, 1996). Available on the Internet at: http://www.who.int/msa/mnh/ems/dalys/intro.htm. Cited in U.S. Department of Health and Human Services, "Mental health: A Report of the Surgeon General, Executive Summary" (Rockville, Md.: U.S. Department of Health and Human Services, Substance Abuse and Mental Health Services Administration, Center for Mental Health Services, National Institutes of Health, National Institute of Mental Health, 1999): ix.

2. C. J. L. Murray, and A. D. Lopez, eds., *Summary: The Global Burden of Disease: A Comprehensive Assessment of Mortality and Disability from Diseases, Injuries, and Risk Factors in 1990 and Projected to 2020* (Cambridge: Harvard School of Public Health on Behalf of the World Health Organization and the World Bank, Harvard University Press, 1996). Available on the Internet at: http://www.who.int/msa/mnh/ems/dalys/intro.htm.

3. R. C. Kessler, et al., "A methodology for estimating the 12-month prevalence of serious mental illness," in: R. W. Manderscheid and M. J. Henderson, eds., *Mental Health, United*

States, 1999 (Rockville, Md.: Center for Mental Health Services, 1998): 99–109.

4. Center for Mental Health Services, *Survey of Mental Health Organizations and General Mental Health Services* (Rockville, Md.: Center for Mental Health Services, 1998).

5. Elizabeth Carla Jacobs, M.D., and Beth Howard, eds., L.P.S., "A New Vision for Mental Health Treatment Laws: A Report by the LPS Reform Task Force," published by the LPS Reform Task Force, Long Beach, California (March 1999): 32–3. The L.P.S. is the Lanterman Petris Short Act, passed in 1967, which closed the doors of many mental hospitals and drastically reduced the staff in many others.

6. The numbers are likely higher today. This was the estimated cost in 1990, the most recent year for which estimates are available, according to "Mental Health: A Report of the U.S. Surgeon General" (1999); available on the Internet at
http://www.surgeongeneral.gov/library/mentalhealth/chapter6/sec2.html#figure6_3. D. P. Rice and L. S. Miller, "The economic burden of schizophrenia: conceptual and methodological issues, and cost estimates," in M. Moscarelli, A. Rupp, and N. Sartorius, eds., *Handbook of Mental Health Economics and Health Policy: Schizophrenia, Vol. 1* (New York: John Wiley and Sons, 1996): 321–4.

7. The full text of the letter is available on the Internet at: http://www.connix.com/~narpa/mosher.htm.

1: What Is Schizophrenia, and Who Suffers from It?

8. NIMH, "Schizophrenia," National Institute of Mental Health (NIH Publication No. 99-3517); available on the Internet at: http://www.nimh.nih.gov/publicat/schizoph.cfm. Irving I. Gottesman, *Schizophrenia Genesis: The Origins of Madness* (New York: W. H. Freeman and Company, 1991): xi.

9. *Taber's Cyclopedic Medical Dictionary,* 17th ed. (Philadelphia: F. A. Davis Company, 1993): 1759.

10. Irving I. Gottesman, *Schizophrenia Genesis: The Origins of Madness* (New York: W. H. Freeman and Company, 1991): 8.

11. Richard S. E. Keefe and Philip D. Harvey, *Understanding Schizophrenia: A Guide to the New Research on Causes and Treatment* (New York: Free Press/Simon & Schuster, 1994): 10.

12. Sources for statistics: American Psychiatric Association, *DSM-IV-TR (Diagnostic and Statistical Manual of Mental Disorders, 4th Edition, Text Revision)* (Washington: American Psychiatric Association, 2000): 304, 307–8. *Masks of Madness: Science of Healing,* a film written, produced, and directed by Connie Bortnick, produced in association with the Canadian Schizophrenia Foundation, 16 Florence Avenue, Toronto, Ontario M2N 1E9 Canada (Sisyphus Communications, Ltd., 1998). NAMI, "Untreated Mental Illness: A Needless Human Tragedy," Omnibus Mental Illness Recovery Act (OMIRA) Brochure, published by NAMI (National Alliance for the Mentally Ill), available at their website: www.nami.org. NARSAD, "Understanding Schizophrenia: A Guide for People with Schizophrenia and Their Families," 1996, NARSAD (National Alliance for Research on Schizophrenia and Depression), 60 Cutter Mill Road, Great Neck, NY 11021; (800) 829-8289 or (516) 829-0091; website: http://www.mhsource.com/narsad.html. NIMH, "Schizophrenia," National Institute of Mental Health (NIH Publication No. 99-3517); available on the Internet at: http://www.nimh.nih.gov/publicat/schizoph.cfm. E. Fuller Torrey, M.D., *Surviving Schizophrenia: A Manual for Families, Consumers, and Providers* (New York: HarperPerennial, 1995): 215.

13. *Autobiography of a Schizophrenic Girl: The True Story of "Renée"* (New York: Meridian/Penguin, 1994): 26.

14. Ibid., 98.

15. *DSM-IV-TR* 304.

16. Abram Hoffer, M.D., Ph.D., and Humphry Osmond, M.R.C.S., D.P.M., *How to Live with Schizophrenia* (New York: Citadel Press/Carol Publishing, 1992): 27.

17. *DSM-IV-TR* 301.

18. E. Fuller Torrey, M.D., *Surviving Schizophrenia: A Manual for Families, Consumers, and Providers* (New York: HarperPerennial, 1995): 39, 40.

19. David A. Kahn, M.D., et al., "Treatment of Bipolar Disorder: A Guide for Patients and Families," A Postgraduate Medicine Special Report, April 2000; available from NDMDA (National Depressive and Manic-Depressive Association), tel: 800-826-3632, website: www.ndmda.org; or NAMI (National Alliance for the Mentally Ill), tel: 800-950-6264, website: www.nami.org.

20. *DSM-IV-TR* 304.

21. *DSM-IV-TR* 312

22. Abram Hoffer, M.D., Ph.D., and Humphry Osmond, M.R.C.S., D.P.M., *How to Live with Schizophrenia* (New York: Citadel Press/Carol Publishing, 1992): 27.

23. *DSM-IV-TR* 313.

24. *DSM-IV-TR* 314.

25. From the film *Masks of Madness: Science of Healing,* written, produced, and directed by Connie Bortnick, produced in association with the Canadian Schizophrenic Foundation, 16 Florence Avenue, Toronto, Ontario M2N 1E9 Canada (Sisyphus Communications, Ltd., 1998).

26. Francis Mark Mondimore, M.D., *Bipolar Disorder: A Guide for Patients and Families* (Baltimore, Md.: John Hopkins University Press, 1999): 51.

27. Richard S. E. Keefe and Philip D. Harvey, *Understanding Schizophrenia: A Guide to the New Research on Causes and Treatment* (New York: Free Press/Simon & Schuster, 1994): 61.

28. Irving I. Gottesman, *Schizophrenia Genesis: The Origins of Madness* (New York: W. H. Freeman and Company, 1991): 80–81. E. Fuller Torrey, M.D., *Surviving Schizophrenia: A Manual for Families, Consumers, and Providers* (New York: HarperPerennial, 1995): 12–13.

29. E. Fuller Torrey, M.D., *Surviving Schizophrenia: A Manual for Families, Consumers, and Providers* (New York: HarperPerennial, 1995): 14–15.

30. *DSM-IV-TR* 307.

31. Peter R. Breggin, M.D., and David Cohen, Ph.D., *Your Drug May Be Your Problem: How and Why to Stop Taking Psychiatric Medications* (Reading, Mass.: Perseus Books, 1999): 41.

32. Torrey, *Surviving Schizophrenia,* 7–8.

33. Richard S. E. Keefe and Philip D. Harvey, *Understanding Schizophrenia: A Guide to the New Research on Causes and Treatment* (New York: Free Press/Simon & Schuster, 1994): 54.

34. *DSM-IV-TR* 308.

35. NIMH, "Schizophrenia," National Institute of Mental Health (NIH Publication No. 99-3517); available on the Internet at: http://www.nimh.nih.gov/publicat/schizoph.cfm.

36. Keefe and Harvey, *Understanding Schizophrenia,* 47.

37. *DSM-IV-TR* 304.

38. NARSAD, "Fact Sheet: The Warning Signs of Suicide," NARSAD (National Alliance for Research on Schizophrenia and Depression), 60 Cutter Mill Road, Suite 404, Great Neck, NY 11021; tel: (516) 829-0091; fax: (516) 487-6930; website: www.narsad.org.

39. *DSM-IV-TR* 304.

40. Rita Elkins, *Depression and Natural Medicine: A Nutritional Approach to Depression and Mood Swings* (Pleasant Grove, Utah: Woodland Publishing, 1995): 16. Demitri Papolos, M.D., and Janice Papolos, *Overcoming Depression: The Definitive Resource for Patients and Families Who Live with Depression and Manic-Depression* (New York: HarperPerennial, 1997): 270.

41. *DSM-IV-TR* 309.

42. E. Fuller Torrey, M.D., *Surviving Schizophrenia: A Manual for Families, Consumers, and Providers* (New York: HarperPerennial, 1995): 122.

43. Ibid.

44. Kay Redfield Jamison, *Touched with Fire: Manic-Depressive Illness and the Artistic Temperament* (New York: Free Press/Simon & Schuster, 1993): 249.

45. E. Fuller Torrey, M.D., *Surviving Schizophrenia: A Manual for Families, Consumers, and Providers* (New York: HarperPerennial, 1995): 123.

46. Irving I. Gottesman, *Schizophrenia Genesis: The Origins of Madness* (New York: W.H. Freeman and Company, 1991): 9.

47. Demitri Papolos, M.D., and Janice Papolos, *Overcoming Depression: The Definitive Resource for Patients and Families Who Live with Depression and Manic-Depression* (New York: HarperPerennial, 1997): 32–33.

48. Catherine Carrigan, *Healing Depression: A Holistic Guide* (New York: Marlowe and Company, 2000): 75.

49. Irving I. Gottesman, *Schizophrenia Genesis: The Origins of Madness* (New York: W.H. Freeman and Company, 1991): 64.

50. E. Fuller Torrey, M.D., *Surviving Schizophrenia: A Manual for Families, Consumers, and Providers* (New York: HarperPerennial, 1995): 24.

51. Elizabeth Carla Jacobs, M.D., and Beth Howard, eds., "A New Vision for Mental Health Treatment Laws: A Report by the LPS Reform Task Force," published by the LPS Reform Task Force, Long Beach, California (March 1999): 32–33.

52. *Masks of Madness: Science of Healing,* a film written, produced, and directed by Connie Bortnick, produced in association with the Canadian Schizophrenia Foundation, 16 Florence Avenue, Toronto, Ontario M2N 1E9 Canada (Sisyphus Communications, Ltd., 1998).

53. "Untreated Mental Illness: A Needless Human Tragedy," Omnibus Mental Illness Recovery Act (OMIRA) Brochure, published by NAMI (National Alliance for the Mentally Ill), available at their website: www.nami.org.

54. Ron Honberg, "Weston Case Raises Legal Questions Over Forced Medication," available on the NAMI (National Alliance for the Mentally Ill) website at: http://www.nami.org/legal/990828b.html.

55. Jay Neugeboren, *Imagining Robert: My Brother, Madness, and Survival—A Memoir* (New York: Henry Holt, 1997): 4.

56. Patty Duke and Gloria Hochman, *A Brilliant Madness: Living with Manic-Depressive Illness* (New York: Bantam, 1993): 205.

57. Richard S. E. Keefe and Philip D. Harvey, *Understanding Schizophrenia: A Guide to the New Research on Causes and Treatment* (New York: Free Press/Simon & Schuster, 1994): 108–9.

58. Eva Edelman, *Natural Healing for Schizophrenia and Other Common Mental Disorders,* 3d ed. (Eugene, Ore.: Borage Books, 2001): 142.

59. Joseph Glenmullen, M.D., *Prozac Backlash* (New York: Touchstone/Simon & Schuster, 2000): 16.

60. E. C. Azmitia and P. M. Whitaker-Azmitia, "Awakening the sleeping giant: anatomy and plasticity of the brain serotonergic system," *Journal of Clinical Psychiatry* 52:12 suppl. (1991): 4–16. Cited in Joseph Glenmullen, M.D., *Prozac Backlash* (New York: Touchstone/Simon & Schuster, 2000): 16.

61. Glenmullen, *Prozac Backlash,* 340.

62. *Taber's Cyclopedic Medical Dictionary,* 17th ed. (Philadelphia: F. A. Davis Company, 1993): 662, 1318.

63. Edelman, *Natural Healing for Schizophrenia,* 142.

64. Russell Jaffe, M.D., Ph.D., and Oscar Rogers Kruesi, M.D., "The biochemical-immunity window: a molecular view of psychiatric case management," *Journal of Applied Nutrition* 44:2 (1992).

65. Edelman, *Natural Healing for Schizophrenia,* 145.

66. Peter R. Breggin, M.D., and David Cohen, Ph.D., *Your Drug May Be Your Problem: How and Why to Stop Taking Psychiatric Medications* (Reading, Mass.: Perseus Books, 1999): 76, 77.

67. NIMH, "Schizophrenia," National Institute of Mental Health (NIH Publication No. 99-3517); available on the Internet at: http://www.nimh.nih.gov/publicat/schizoph.cfm.

68. John F. Thornton, et al., "Schizophrenia: The Medications," available on the Internet at: http://www.mentalhealth.com/book/p42-sc3.html#Head_5.

69. Ibid.

70. Peter R. Breggin, M.D., and David Cohen, Ph.D., *Your Drug May Be Your Problem: How and Why to Stop Taking Psychiatric Medications* (Reading, Mass.: Perseus Books, 1999): 78.

71. Personal communication with Dr. Rimland, 2002. Also cited in Edelman, *Natural Healing for Schizophrenia,* 147.

72. M. Jarema and M. Kuciska, "Practical aspects of drug resistance in schizophrenia," *Psychiatria Polska* 34:5 (September-October 2000): 721–40.

73. "New Treatments for Schizophrenia," *Harvard Mental Health Letter* 14:10 (April 1998); available as Pamphlet 2 of the Publications of the World Fellowship for Schizophrenia and Allied Disorders, 869 Yonge Street, Suite 104, Toronto, Ontario M4W 2H2, Canada; tel: (416) 961-2855; website: www.world-schizophrenia.org. NIMH, "Schizophrenia," National Institute of Mental Health (NIH Publication No. 99-3517); available on the Internet at: http://www.nimh.nih.gov/publicat/schizoph.cfm.

74. "New Treatments for Schizophrenia," *Harvard Mental Health Letter* 14:10 (April 1998); available as Pamphlet 2 of the Publications of the World Fellowship for Schizophrenia and Allied Disorders, 869 Yonge Street, Suite 104, Toronto, Ontario M4W 2H2, Canada; tel: (416) 961-2855; website: www.world-schizophrenia.org.

75. C. S. Brown, et al., "Atypical antipsychotics: Part II: Adverse effects, drug interactions, and costs," *Annals of Pharmacotherapy* 33:2 (February 1999): 210–217. Peter R. Breggin, M.D., and David Cohen, Ph.D., *Your Drug May Be Your Problem: How and Why to Stop Taking Psychiatric Medications* (Reading, Mass.: Perseus Books, 1999): 47.

76. G. Remington and S. Kapur, "Atypical antipsychotics: Are some more atypical than others?" *Psychopharmacology* 148:1 (January 2000): 3–15.

77. J. Geddes, et al., "Atypical antipsychotics in the treatment of schizophrenia: Systematic overview and meta-regression analysis," *British Medical Journal* 321:7273 (December 2, 2000): 1371–76.

78. "Surge in Anti-Psychotic Drugs Given to Kids Draws Concern," *USA Today* (July 23, 2002); available on the Internet at: http://www.healthyplace.com/Communities/Thought_Disorders/sc hizo/news/kids-antipsychotics.htm

79. "Depression drugs widely prescribed to children," *Health Watch* 4:2 (June 30, 1999): 2.

80. Joseph Glenmullen, M.D., *Prozac Backlash* (New York: Touchstone/Simon & Schuster, 2000). Peter R. Breggin, M.D., and David Cohen, Ph.D., *Your Drug May Be Your Problem: How and Why to Stop Taking Psychiatric Medications* (Reading, Mass.: Perseus Books, 1999): 46–47.

81. Peter R. Breggin, M.D., and David Cohen, Ph.D., *Your Drug May Be Your Problem: How and Why to Stop Taking Psychiatric Medications* (Reading, Mass.: Perseus Books, 1999): 82–83.

2: Causes, Triggers, and Contributors

82. Quoted on the website of Volunteers in Psychotherapy, in an article entitled "Are Personal and Emotional Problems Diseases?" available on the Internet at www.ctvip.org/web2c.html, or contact Richard Shulman, Ph.D., director, Volunteers In Psychotherapy, Inc., 7 South Main Street, West Hartford, CT 06107; tel: (860) 233-5115.

83. Ibid.

84. Ibid.

85. Joseph Glenmullen, M.D., *Prozac Backlash* (New York: Touchstone/Simon & Schuster, 2000): 193.

86. U.S. Department of Health and Human Services, "Mental Health: A Report of the Surgeon General, Executive Summary," (Rockville, Md.: U.S. Department of Health and Human Services, Substance Abuse and Mental Health Services Administration, Center for Mental Health Services, National Institutes of Health, National Institute of Mental Health, 1999): x.

87. Joseph Glenmullen, M.D., *Prozac Backlash* (New York: Touchstone/Simon & Schuster, 2000): 198.

88. NARSAD, "Understanding Schizophrenia: A Guide for People with Schizophrenia and Their Families," 1996, NARSAD (National Alliance for Research on Schizophrenia and Depression), 60 Cutter Mill Road, Great Neck, NY 11021; (800) 829-8289 or (516) 829-0091; website: http://www.mhsource.com/narsad.html.

89. Irving I. Gottesman, *Schizophrenia Genesis: The Origins of Madness* (New York: W. H. Freeman and Company, 1991): 102–103.

90. Richard S. E. Keefe and Philip D. Harvey, *Understanding Schizophrenia: A Guide to the New Research on Causes and Treatment* (New York: Free Press/Simon & Schuster, 1994): 99.

91. Richard Leviton, *The Healthy Living Space* (Charlottesville, Va.: Hampton Roads, 2001): 2.

92. Ibid., 3.

93. "Doctors warn developmental disabilities epidemic from toxins," LDA (Learning Disabilities Association of America) *Newsbriefs* 35:4 (July/August 2000): 3–5; executive summary from the report by the Greater Boston Physicians for Social Responsibility, "In Harm's Way—Toxic Threats to Child Development," available at http://www.igc.org/psr/ihw.htm; for LDA, http://www.ldanatl.org.

94. Philip J. Landrigan, *Environmental Neurotoxicology* (Washington: National Academy Press, 1992): 2; cited in Richard Leviton, *The Healthy Living Space* (Charlottesville, Va.: Hampton Roads, 2001): 13.

95. Sherry A. Rogers, M.D., *Depression—Cured at Last!* (Sarasota, Fla.: SK Publishing, 1997): 94.

96. John Foster, M.D., "Is depression natural in an unnatural world?" *Well-Being Journal* (Spring 2001): 11; website: www.wellbeingjournal.com.

97. Eva Edelman, *Natural Healing for Schizophrenia and Other Common Mental Disorders*, 3d ed. (Eugene, Ore.: Borage Books, 2001): 93.

98. Dietrich Klinghardt, M.D., Ph.D., "Amalgam/Mercury Detox as a Treatment for Chronic Viral, Bacterial, and Fungal Illnesses," lecture presented at the Annual Meeting of the International and American Academy of Clinical Nutrition, San Diego, Calif., September 1996.

99. Morton Walker, D.P.M., *Elements of Danger: Protect Yourself Against the Hazards of Modern Dentistry* (Charlottesville, Va.: Hampton Roads, 2000): 138, 141.

100. Edelman, *Natural Healing for Schizophrenia,* 93.

101. Syd Baumel, *Dealing with Depression Naturally* (Los Angeles: Keats Publishing, 2000): 34.

102. Edelman, *Natural Healing for Schizophrenia,* 96.

103. D. P. Perl and A. R. Bordy, "Detection of aluminum by semi-x-ray spectrometry with neurofibrillary tangle-bearing neurons of Alzheimer's disease," *Neurotox* (1990): 133–7. Morton Walker, D.P.M., *Elements of Danger: Protect Yourself Against the Hazards of Modern Dentistry* (Charlottesville, Va.: Hampton Roads, 2000): 218–9. Edelman, *Natural Healing for Schizophrenia,* 98.

104. See "Depression: Causes" (Food Allergies/Intolerances) at http://www.yournutrition.co.uk/specific_health_problems_D.htm.

105. Devi S. Nambudripad, D.C., L.Ac., R.N., Ph.D., *Say Goodbye to Illness, New & Revised edition* (Buena Park, Calif.: Delta Publishing, 1999): 35.

106. Ibid., 33.

107. Ibid.

108. C. C. Pfeiffer, *Nutrition and Mental Illness* (Rochester, Vt.: Healing Arts Press, 1987).

109. "New evidence points to opioids," *Autism Research Review International* 5:4 (1991).

110. Paul Shattock, "Urinary Peptides and Associated Metabolites in the Urine of People with Autism Spectrum Disorders," syllabus material for the main DAN! lecture at the DAN! (Defeat Autism Now!) 2000 Conference, in the conference booklet: 79–83; published by the Autism Research Institute in San Diego, Calif. (fax: 619-563-6840 or website: www.autism.com/ari). "New

evidence points to opioids," *Autism Research Review International* 5:4 (1991). A. J. Wakefield, et al., "Ileal-lymphoid-nodular hyperplasia, non-specific colitis, and pervasive developmental disorder in children," *Lancet* 351 (February 28, 1998): 637–41.

111. C. Hallert, et al., "Psychic disturbances in adult coeliac disease III. Reduced central monoamine metabolism and signs of depression," *Scandinavian Journal of Gastroenterology* 17 (1982): 25–8.

112. See "Depression: Causes" (Food Allergies/Intolerances) at http://www.yournutrition.co.uk/specific_health_problems_D.htm.

113. Adapted from: Karyn Seroussi, *Unraveling the Mystery of Autism and Pervasive Developmental Disorder* (New York: Simon & Schuster, 2000) 229–30.

114. Sherry A. Rogers, M.D., *Depression—Cured at Last!* (Sarasota, Fla.: SK Publishing, 1997): 460.

115. Ibid., 461–62.

116. Eva Edelman, *Natural Healing for Schizophrenia and Other Common Mental Disorders*, 3d ed. (Eugene, Ore.: Borage Books, 2001): 108.

117. Rogers, *Depression,* 165–67.

118. Rogers, *Depression,* 166.

119. Personal communication with Dr. Rau, 2001.

120. John N. Hathcock, *Nutritional Toxicology, Vol. I* (New York: Academic Press, 1982): 462. L. D. Stegink and L. J. Filer, Jr., eds., *Aspartame* (New York: Marcel Dekker, 1984): 350, 359. Bryan Ballantyne, Timothy Marrs, and Paul Turner, eds., *General and Applied Toxicology, Vol. 1* (New York: Stockton Press, 1993): 482.

121. Leon Chaitow, *Thorson's Guide to Amino Acids* (London: Thorson, 1991): 95.

122. Susan C. Smolinske, *Handbook of Food, Drug, and Cosmetic Excipients* (Boca Raton, Fla.: CRC Press, 1992): 236.

123. Bernard Rimland, Ph.D., "The Feingold diet: An assessment of the reviews by Marttes, by Kavale and Forness and others," *Journal of Learning Disabilities* 16:6 (June/July 1983): 331. (Available from the Autism Research Institute, Publication #51.)

124. Hyman J. Roberts, "Reactions attributed to aspartame containing products: 551 cases," *Natural Food & Farming* (March 1992): 23–28.

125. Katherine S. Rowe and Kenneth J. Rowe, "Synthetic food coloring and behavior: A dose response effect in a double-blind, placebo-controlled, repeated-measures study," *Journal of Pediatrics* (November 1994): 691–98, in "Color me hyperactive," *Autism Research Review International* 9:2 (1995).

126. Richard A. Kunin, M.D., "Principles That Identify Orthormolecular Medicine: A Unique Medical Specialty," available on the Internet at: http://www.orthomed.org/kunin.htm.

127. Claudio Galli and Artemis P. Simopoulos, eds., *Dietary W3 and W6 Fatty Acids: Biological Effects and Nutritional Essentiality* (New York: Kluwer/Plenum, 1989). Claudio Galli and Artemis P. Simopoulos, *Effects of Fatty Acids and Lipids in Health and Disease* (New York: S. Karger, 1994). Joseph Mercola, "Where's the Real Beef?" available on the Internet at www.mercola.com/beef/main.htm.

128. Presenter statement by Andrew Stoll, M.D., in the DAN! (Defeat Autism Now!) 2000 Conference booklet: 8; published by the Autism Research Institute in San Diego, Calif. (fax: 619-563-6840 or website: www.autism.com/ari).

129. M. A. Crawford, A. G. Hassam, and P. A. Stevens, "Essential fatty acid requirements in pregnancy and lactation with special reference to brain development," *Progress in Lipid Research* 20 (1981): 31–40.

130. "Healing mood disorders with essential fatty acids," *Doctors' Prescription for Healthy Living* 4:6, 1.

131. M. P. Freeman, "Omega-3 fatty acids in psychiatry: A review," *Annals of Clinical Psychiatry* 12:3 (September 2000): 159–65.

132. J. D. E. Laugherne, et al., "Fatty acids and schizophrenia," *Lipids* 31: suppl (1996), S163–S165.

133. Irving I. Gottesman, *Schizophrenia Genesis: The Origins of Madness* (New York: W. H. Freeman and Company, 1991): 61–2.

134. Eva Edelman, *Natural Healing for Schizophrenia and Other Common Mental Disorders*, 3d ed. (Eugene, Ore.: Borage Books, 2001): 26.

135. E. H. Cook and B. L. Leventhal, "The serotonin system in autism," *Current Opinions in Pediatrics* 8:4 (August 1996): 348–54.

136. Richard S. E. Keefe and Philip D. Harvey, *Understanding Schizophrenia: A Guide to the New Research on Causes and Treatment* (New York: Free Press/Simon & Schuster, 1994): 128.

137. *DSM-IV-TR* 305.

138. E. Fuller Torrey, M.D., et al., *Schizophrenia and Manic-Depressive Disorder: The Biological Roots of Mental Illness as Revealed by the Landmark Study of Identical Twins* (New York: Basic Books, 1994): 64.

139. *DSM-IV-TR* 305. E. Fuller Torrey, et al., "Birth seasonality in bipolar disorder, schizophrenia, schizoaffective disorder, and still-births," *Schizophrenia Research 21* (1996): 141–9.

140. E. Fuller Torrey, M.D., *Surviving Schizophrenia: A Manual for Families, Consumers, and Providers* (New York: HarperPerennial, 1995): 154.

141. Richard S. E. Keefe and Philip D. Harvey, *Understanding Schizophrenia: A Guide to the New Research on Causes and Treatment* (New York: Free Press/Simon & Schuster, 1994): 94.

142. E. Fuller Torrey, M.D., *Surviving Schizophrenia: A Manual for Families, Consumers, and Providers* (New York: HarperPerennial, 1995): 116, 117.

143. Eva Edelman, *Natural Healing for Schizophrenia and Other Common Mental Disorders*, 3d ed. (Eugene, Ore.: Borage Books, 2001): 70.

144. Ibid., 70.

145. Syd Baumel, *Dealing with Depression Naturally* (Los Angeles: Keats Publishing, 2000): 12.

146. Ronald Hoffman, "Beyond Prozac: Natural therapies for anxiety and depression," *Innovation: The Health Letter of FAIM* (January 31, 1999): 10–11, 13, 15, 17, 19.

147. Peter C. Whybrow, M.D., *A Mood Apart: The Thinker's Guide to Emotion and Its Disorders* (New York: HarperPerennial, 1997): 212.

148. *DSM-IV-TR* 309.

149. Nic Rowan, "Estrogen May Help Schizophrenic Women," Reuters Health Information (March 13, 2001); available on the Internet at: www.nlm.nih.gov/medlineplus/news/fullstory_669.html.

150. *DSM-IV-TR* 309, 334.

151. *DSM-IV-TR* 339.

152. *DSM-IV-TR* 340–41.

153. Anne Harding, "Antidepressants Hazardous for Some Mentally Ill," Reuters Health Information (March 20, 2001); available

on the Internet at: http://www.nlm.nih.gov/medlineplus/news/full story_832.html.

154. NIMH, "Schizophrenia," National Institute of Mental Health (NIH Publication No. 99-3517); available on the Internet at: http://www.nimh.nih.gov/publicat/schizoph.cfm.

155. Richard S. E. Keefe and Philip D. Harvey, *Understanding Schizophrenia: A Guide to the New Research on Causes and Treatment* (New York: Free Press/Simon & Schuster, 1994): 47.

156. E. Fuller Torrey, M.D., *Surviving Schizophrenia: A Manual for Families, Consumers, and Providers* (New York: HarperPerennial, 1995): 257.

157. Rita Elkins, *Depression and Natural Medicine: A Nutritional Approach to Depression and Mood Swings* (Pleasant Grove, Utah: Woodland Publishing, 1995): 138.

158. Ibid.

159. Ibid. Eva Edelman, *Natural Healing for Schizophrenia and Other Common Mental Disorders*, 3d ed. (Eugene, Ore.: Borage Books, 2001): 85.

160. Edelman, *Natural Healing for Schizophrenia*, 86.

161. Richard S. E. Keefe and Philip D. Harvey, *Understanding Schizophrenia: A Guide to the New Research on Causes and Treatment* (New York: Free Press/Simon & Schuster, 1994): 47.

162. E. Fuller Torrey, M.D., *Surviving Schizophrenia: A Manual for Families, Consumers, and Providers* (New York: HarperPerennial, 1995): 252.

163. Ibid.

164. Edelman, *Natural Healing for Schizophrenia*, 84.

165. Edelman, *Natural Healing for Schizophrenia*, 134.

166. Rita Elkins, *Depression and Natural Medicine: A Nutritional Approach to Depression and Mood Swings* (Pleasant Grove, Utah: Woodland Publishing, 1995): 103. Edelman, 40.

167. M. E. McGrath, *Schizophrenia Bulletin* 10 (1984): 638–40. Cited in Irving I. Gottesman, *Schizophrenia Genesis: The Origins of Madness* (New York: W. H. Freeman and Company, 1991): 42.

168. David Kaiser, M.D., "Not by Chemicals Alone: A Hard Look at Psychiatric Medicine," available on the Internet at: www.rust.net/~norman/kaiser.html.

169. Richard S. E. Keefe and Philip D. Harvey, *Understanding Schizophrenia: A Guide to the New Research on Causes and Treatment* (New York: Free Press/Simon & Schuster, 1994): 175.

170. M. J. Goldstein, et al., "Drug and family therapy in the aftercare of acute schizophrenia," *Archives of General Psychiatry* 45 (1988): 225–31.

3: Orthomolecular Psychiatry

171. From the film *Masks of Madness: Science of Healing,* written, produced, and directed by Connie Bortnick, produced in association with the Canadian Schizophrenia Foundation, 16 Florence Avenue, Toronto, Ontario M2N 1E9 Canada (Sisyphus Communications, Ltd., 1998).

172. A. Hoffer and Ms. J.M., "Inside schizophrenia: before and after treatment," *Journal of Orthomolecular Medicine* 11:1 (1996): 7–37; available on the Internet at:
http://www.orthomed.org/links/papers/hofshz2.htm.

173. Abram Hoffer, "Gaining control of schizophrenia," *American Journal of Natural Medicine* 5:5 (June 30, 1998): 21–25.

174. Abram Hoffer, M.D., Ph.D., *Orthomolecular Treatment for Schizophrenia* (Los Angeles: Keats Publishing, 1999): 7.

175. Abram Hoffer, "Chronic schizophrenic patients treated ten years or more," *Journal of Orthomolecular Medicine* 9:1 (1994): 7–37; available on the Internet at: http://www.orthomed.org/links/papers/hofschz.htm.

176. Abram Hoffer, "Gaining control of schizophrenia," *American Journal of Natural Medicine* 5:5 (June 30, 1998): 21–25.

177. From the film *Masks of Madness: Science of Healing,* written, produced, and directed by Connie Bortnick, produced in association with the Canadian Schizophrenia Foundation, 16 Florence Avenue, Toronto, Ontario M2N 1E9 Canada (Sisyphus Communications, Ltd., 1998).

178. Ibid.

179. Abram Hoffer, M.D., Ph.D., *Orthomolecular Treatment for Schizophrenia* (Los Angeles: Keats Publishing, 1999): 24–25.

180. Abram Hoffer, "Gaining control of schizophrenia," *American Journal of Natural Medicine* 5:5 (June 30, 1998): 21–25. Abram Hoffer, M.D., Ph.D., and Humphry Osmond, M.R.C.S.,

D.P.M., *How to Live with Schizophrenia* (New York: Citadel Press/ Carol Publishing, 1992): 172.

181. From the film *Masks of Madness: Science of Healing*, written, produced, and directed by Connie Bortnick, produced in association with the Canadian Schizophrenia Foundation, 16 Florence Avenue, Toronto, Ontario M2N 1E9 Canada (Sisyphus Communications, Ltd., 1998).

182. Ibid.

183. Abram Hoffer, M.D., Ph.D., *Orthomolecular Treatment for Schizophrenia* (Los Angeles: Keats Publishing, 1999): 19–20.

184. From the film *Masks of Madness: Science of Healing*, written, produced, and directed by Connie Bortnick, produced in association with the Canadian Schizophrenia Foundation, 16 Florence Avenue, Toronto, Ontario M2N 1E9 Canada (Sisyphus Communications, Ltd., 1998).

185. Abram Hoffer, M.D., Ph.D., and Humphry Osmond, M.R.C.S., D.P.M., *How to Live with Schizophrenia* (New York: Citadel Press/Carol Publishing, 1992): 175.

186. From the film *Masks of Madness: Science of Healing*, written, produced, and directed by Connie Bortnick, produced in association with the Canadian Schizophrenia Foundation, 16 Florence Avenue, Toronto, Ontario M2N 1E9 Canada (Sisyphus Communications, Ltd., 1998).

187. Abram Hoffer, "Gaining control of schizophrenia," *American Journal of Natural Medicine* 5:5 (June 30, 1998): 21–25.

188. Michael Lesser, M.D., *The Brain Chemistry Diet* (New York: Putnam, 2002).

189. Michael Lesser, M.D., *Nutrition and Vitamin Therapy* (New York: Bantam, 1981): 42.

190. H. Vanderkamp, "A biochemical abnormality in schizophrenia involving ascorbic acid," *International Journal of Neurochemistry and Psychiatry* 2 (1966): 204–6.

191. Michael Lesser, M.D., *Nutrition and Vitamin Therapy* (New York: Bantam, 1981): 46.

192. Abram Hoffer, "Gaining control of schizophrenia," *American Journal of Natural Medicine* 5:5 (June 30, 1998): 21–25.

193. Ibid.

194. Ibid.

195. Abram Hoffer, M.D., Ph.D., *Orthomolecular Treatment for Schizophrenia* (Los Angeles: Keats Publishing, 1999): 26.

196. Abram Hoffer, M.D., Ph.D., and Humphry Osmond, M.R.C.S., D.P.M., *How to Live with Schizophrenia* (New York: Citadel Press/Carol Publishing, 1992): 16, 90.

197. From the film *Masks of Madness: Science of Healing,* written, produced, and directed by Connie Bortnick, produced in association with the Canadian Schizophrenia Foundation, 16 Florence Avenue, Toronto, Ontario M2N 1E9 Canada (Sisyphus Communications, Ltd., 1998).

198. Abram Hoffer, M.D., Ph.D., *Orthomolecular Treatment for Schizophrenia* (Los Angeles: Keats Publishing, 1999): 12.

199. From the film *Masks of Madness: Science of Healing,* written, produced, and directed by Connie Bortnick, produced in association with the Canadian Schizophrenia Foundation, 16 Florence Avenue, Toronto, Ontario M2N 1E9 Canada (Sisyphus Communications, Ltd., 1998).

200. Abram Hoffer, "Gaining control of schizophrenia," *American Journal of Natural Medicine* 5:5 (June 30, 1998): 21–25.

4: Biochemical Treatment of Schizophrenia

201. William J. Walsh, Ph.D., "Biochemical treatment: medicines for the next century," *NOHA (Nutrition for Optimal Health Association) News* 16:3 (Summer 1991), available on the HRI-PTC Website (www.hriptc.org/nextcentury.htm).

202. Ibid.

203. From the film *Masks of Madness: Science of Healing,* written, produced, and directed by Connie Bortnick, produced in association with the Canadian Schizophrenia Foundation, 16 Florence Avenue, Toronto, Ontario M2N 1E9 Canada (Sisyphus Communications, Ltd., 1998). To contact the Institute for Optimum Nutrition (ION), Blades Court, Deodar Road, London SW15 2NU England; tel: 020 8877 9993; Fax: 020 8877 9980; website: www.ion.ac.uk.

204. William J. Walsh, Ph.D., "Biochemical treatment: medicines for the next century," *NOHA (Nutrition for Optimal Health Association) News* 16:3 (Summer 1991), available on the HRI-PTC Website (www.hriptc.org/nextcentury.htm). William J. Walsh, Ph.D., "The Critical Role of Nutrients in Severe Mental Symptoms,"

available on the Internet (www.alternativementalhealth.com/articles/article-pffeiffer.htm).

205. William J. Walsh, Ph.D., "Biochemical treatment: Medicines for the next century," *NOHA (Nutrition for Optimal Health Association) News* 16:3 (Summer 1991), available on the HRI-PTC Website (www.hriptc.org/nextcentury.htm).

206. M. E. McGrath, *Schizophrenia Bulletin* 10 (1984): 638–40. Cited in Irving I. Gottesman, *Schizophrenia Genesis: The Origins of Madness* (New York: W. H. Freeman and Company, 1991): 41.

207. Ibid.

5: The Five Levels of Healing

208. E. Fuller Torrey, M.D., *Surviving Schizophrenia: A Manual for Families, Consumers, and Providers* (New York: HarperPerennial, 1995): 123.

209. Stephanie Marohn, *The Natural Medicine Guide to Autism* (Charlottesville, Va.: Hampton Roads, 2002): chapter 5.

210. Richard Leviton, "Migraines, seizures, and mercury toxicity," *Alternative Medicine Digest* 21 (December 1997/January 1998): 61.

6: Restoring the Tempo of Health: Cranial Osteopathy

211. Stephanie Marohn, *The Natural Medicine Guide to Autism* (Charlottesville, Va.: Hampton Roads, 2002): chapter 8.

212. "What Is Osteopathy?" available at the Cranial Academy website (http://www.cranialacademy.org/whatis.html).

213. H.I. Magoun, D.O., *Osteopathy in the Cranial Field,* 3d ed. (Kirksville, Mo.: Journal Printing Company, 1976): 1.

214. "What Is Osteopathy?" available at the Cranial Academy Website (http://www.cranialacademy.org/whatis.html).

215. "Common Problems," available at the Cranial Academy Website (http://www.cranialacademy.org/cmpr.html).

216. Ibid.

217. Ibid.

218. Lawrence Lavine, "Osteopathic and Alternative Medicine Aspects of Autistic Spectrum Disorders," article on the Internet (available at http://trainland.tripod.com/lawrencelavine.htm).

219. Stephanie Marohn, *The Natural Medicine Guide to Autism* (Charlottesville, Va.: Hampton Roads, 2002): chapter 9.

220. Ibid., chapter 8.

221. Anonymous, *Schizophrenia Bulletin* 9 (1983): 439-42. Cited in Irving I. Gottesman, *Schizophrenia Genesis: The Origins of Madness* (New York: W.H. Freeman and Company, 1991): 170.

7: Rebalancing the Vital Force: Homeopathy

222. Personal communication (2001), and Judyth Reichenberg-Ullman, N.D., L.C.S.W., and Robert Ullman, N.D., *Prozac Free: Homeopathic Alternatives to Conventional Drug Therapies* (Berkeley, Calif.: North Atlantic Books, 2002): xiv.

223. Reichenberg-Ullman and Ullman, *Prozac Free,* viii, ix.

224. Reichenberg-Ullman and Ullman, *Prozac Free,* xiv.

225. There is disagreement today over what mental illness Van Gogh had; some professionals say it was schizophrenia, while others say he suffered from bipolar disorder. Quote is from a letter to his brother, Theo, cited in E. Fuller Torrey, M.D., *Surviving Schizophrenia: A Manual for Families, Consumers, and Providers* (New York: HarperPerennial, 1995): 124.

226. Miranda Castro, R.S.Hom., *The Complete Homeopathy Handbook* (New York: St. Martin's Press, 1990): 3–5. Anne Woodham and David Peters, M.D., *Encyclopedia of Healing Therapies* (New York: Dorling Kindersley, 1997): 126.

227. Judyth Reichenberg-Ullman, N.D., M.S.W., and Robert Ullman, N.D., *Ritalin-Free Kids: Safe and Effective Homeopathic Medicine for ADHD, and Other Behavioral and Learning Problems* (Roseville, Calif.: Prima Health, 2000): 83.

228. Ibid., 95.

229. Ibid., 95–96.

230. Personal communication (2001) and Reichenberg-Ullman and Ullman, *Ritalin-Free Kids,* 90.

231. Personal communication (2001) and Reichenberg-Ullman and Ullman, *Prozac Free,* 57, 217–18.

232. Personal communication (2001).

8: Conflict and Spirit: Psychosomatic Medicine

233. *Autobiography of a Schizophrenic Girl: The True Story of "Renee"* (New York: Meridian/Penguin, 1994): 26.

9: The Shamanic View of Mental Illness

234. John Lash, *The Seeker's Handbook* (New York: Harmony Books, 1990): 371.

235. Holger Kalweit, "When Insanity Is a Blessing," in Stanislav Grof, M.D., and Christina Grof, eds., *Spiritual Emergency* (New York: Jeremy P. Tarcher/Putnam, 1989): 80.

236. M. E. McGrath, *Schizophrenia Bulletin* 10 (1984): 638–40. Cited in Irving I. Gottesman, *Schizophrenia Genesis: The Origins of Madness* (New York: W. H. Freeman and Company, 1991): 43.

237. Richard Leviton, *The Healthy Living Space* (Charlottesville, Va.: Hampton Roads, 2001): 354–58.

238. Ibid., 362–63.

239. Ibid., 364.

240. Malidoma Patrice Somé, *Ritual: Power, Healing, and Community* (New York: Penguin, 1997): 12, 19.

241. Malidoma Patrice Somé, *Of Water and the Spirit: Ritual, Magic, and Initiation in the Life of an African Shaman* (New York: Penguin, 1994): 9, 10.

Index

About the Author

Stephanie Marohn has been writing since she was a child. Her adult writing background is extensive in both journalism and non-fiction trade books. In addition to *Natural Medicine First Aid Remedies* and the six books in the Healthy Mind series (*The Natural Medicine Guide to Autism, The Natural Medicine Guide to Depression, The Natural Medicine Guide to Bipolar Disorder, The Natural Medicine Guide to Addiction, The Natural Medicine Guide to Anxiety,* and *The Natural Medicine Guide to Schizophrenia*), she has published more than thirty articles in magazines and newspapers, written two novels and a feature film screenplay, and has had her work included in poetry, prayer, and travel writing anthologies.

Originally from Philadelphia, she has been a resident of the San Francisco Bay Area for over twenty years, and currently lives in Sonoma County, north of the city.

Hampton Roads Publishing Company

. . . for the evolving human spirit

Hampton Roads Publishing Company
publishes books on a variety of subjects,
including metaphysics, health, visionary fiction,
and other related topics.

For a copy of our latest catalog, call toll-free
800-766-8009, or send your name and address to:

Hampton Roads Publishing Company, Inc.
1125 Stoney Ridge Road
Charlottesville, VA 22902

e-mail: hrpc@hrpub.com
www.hrpub.com